the postnatal cookbook

Simple and Nutritious Recipes to Nourish
Your Body and Spirit
during the Fourth Trimester

Jaren Soloff, RD, IBCLC

ULYSSES PRESS

Published in the US by:
ULYSSES PRESS
PO Box 3440
Berkeley, CA 94703
www.ulyssespress.com

ISBN: 978-1-64604-099-5
Library of Congress Control Number: 2020936173

Printed in Korea by Artin Printing Company through We Think
10 9 8 7 6 5 4 3 2 1

Acquisitions editor: Casie Vogel
Managing editor: Claire Chun
Editor: Renee Rutledge
Proofreader: Mark Rhynsburger
Front cover design: Rebecca Lown
Interior design: what!design @ whatweb.com
Interior photos: Jaren Soloff
Interior art: © Le Panda/shutterstock.com

Contents

Introduction

Since you're reading this cookbook you very likely may be a new or expecting mother, or a loved one looking to provide the utmost support and nourishment for a new mother in your life. You are likely no stranger to the importance of nutrition throughout the journey that is pregnancy; however, the period after birth deserves just as much, if not more, attention to nutrition to help you thrive.

"Postnatal" refers to the period immediately after birth, and for the purposes of this cookbook, it is used interchangeably with "postpartum" and "perinatal," which both define the time after childbirth. We are continuing to learn that optimal postnatal nutrition is influenced not just by diet, but by the complex layers that make up physical health, as well as the emotional, social, and cultural support women receive through pregnancy and birth. These factors all contribute to and make up the landscape of a nourishing postpartum.

THE POSTNATAL PERIOD

Pregnancy, birth, and the early days of postpartum are filled with rapid growth, change, and learning. We have learned to support and respect the prenatal period when babies are rapidly developing inside the womb in preparation for the outside world. From choosing the best prenatal vitamins to building a meticulous birth plan, expectant mothers navigate a time that is rife with emotional and physical shifts.

Whether it is their first birth or their fourth, postpartum can take expectant mothers by surprise if they enter into its gates unprepared for the journey ahead. Too often, the primary focus after birth shifts to caring for and nourishing the newborn. Often, mothers are left behind to recover inadequately—physically and emotionally. After birth, an increasing number of women struggle with pelvic floor dysfunction, relational strain, and perinatal mood and anxiety disorders. We simply cannot afford to leave out a plan to nourish mothers after birth.

With this in mind, what is a realistic expectation for recovering from birth, and how can we best support women in preparing for this precious time? While still not collectively defined in terms of length, for many non-Westernized cultures around the globe, several weeks (40 days) is often considered the hallmark of time mothers need to recover from birth and establish breastfeeding. While the terminology may vary depending on the culture, such as "the golden month" in China; "la cuarentana" in Mexico; "sitting in the nest" in Vietnam; and, in the past, a period of "lying in" in the United States, the principle is the same throughout—extended rest. From an anthropological perspective, research has noted that cultures with a social structure that integrates postpartum care have lower incidences of women with postpartum depression.[1] During this time, women from the community, such as mothers and grandmothers, provide special care to support new mothers in replenishing their nutrient stores with special foods and easing up on physically demanding activities. Other women in the family take up the duties of normal life so mothers can focus on nourishing their babies and nurture themselves both physically and emotionally so they have the space to establish breastfeeding.[2]

Another common theme in postpartum care in non-Westernized cultures is confinement, where women have an extended period of rest, are cared for by their mothers or family members, and are cooked nourishing meals to promote healing. This practice of confinement serves not only to relieve new mothers of mundane household tasks but to symbolize that she is being nurtured as she transitions into her new role. Lastly, one of the most distinctly different practices from that of Western cultures is the acknowledgment of a woman's new status as a mother and the honor that goes along with it. Often, these cultures recognize practices such as gift-giving and providing personal care for the mother through social rituals such as washing her hair and feet to show adoration.

In striking contrast to these principles, the current postpartum practices of Westernized culture see postpartum as a race to *bounce back* and *get back to normal* as quickly as possible. In a common hospitalized birth, after the initial recovery from birth, the obstetrician or midwife will pay a brief visit. After this, providers essentially offer no care for women until the six-week medical appointment. At this six-week medical follow-up, women are then evaluated for exercise and sex clearance—however, it is uncommon for a provider to provide support and guidance for common postpartum ailments such as physical healing, nutritional support, or breastfeeding/feeding concerns. At this time, most employers also expect women to return to work. If a woman is lactating, she will now plan and prepare for pumping and storing breastmilk.

This sociocultural background sets the stage for many of the postpartum challenges that increase women's physical and emotional vulnerability. Consider other times in life when our bodies experience an increase in physical demands, such as during an injury or illness, and the support for physical healing, adequate nutrition, and rest that we receive. These essential pieces of postpartum, however, are lacking in the current model of care. Within the modern social climate, the tremendous strides women have made in their career mobility are quickly undercut by messaging that emphasizes a quick return to work and productivity without concern for physical healing or acknowledgment of the transformative process of birth.

What's viewed as the ideal family dynamic places independence over interdependence and, thus, comes at the risk of mothers being more disconnected from networks of support. More often, new families live away from relatives who historically provided the foundation of support to nourish them. The isolation and lack of adequate support can disrupt a mother's physical healing and interrupt the instrumental bonding and nurturing needed for the mother and infant during the first few weeks. Many families know of the adage "it takes a village to raise a child" but lack the connections needed to honor this critical recovery period of postpartum.

If we are going to support optimal outcomes for children and families, we have to work to shift the current framework in Western society toward practices that embody rest, nutrient repletion, and slowing down. While many of us long for an idyllic 40-day resting period, we must also balance these practices with the current cultural dynamic set in place for us.

While Western culture does have a general practice of providing meals for those who have welcomed a newborn into their home, a mother's true postpartum healing and repletion cannot be completed with food alone. In order to assist women in healing, we not only have to provide support with the sometimes mundane tasks of cooking, cleaning, and infant care, we also have to make space to allow women to rest, recover, and heal.

The Postnatal Cookbook proposes a middle path whereby we can integrate postpartum nutrition practices in a manner that does not require exhausting recipes or extensive chopping and preparing, but rather a simple whole-foods approach to healing and creating a postpartum experience that nourishes mind, body, and soul.

Chapter 1

Postnatal Nutrition

To further support the healing needed during the postpartum period, we first need to continue to understand the unique variables that women face during this time period and investigate just how long these variables continue to impact them after they give birth. To date, while many clinicians and health-care providers understand there is a level of physical healing to achieve postpartum, they offer virtually no nutritional support during this time other than the advice that women who are lactating will likely experience an increase in hunger. Even less is known about the differentiation between women who lactate and those who are non-lactating and identifying the unique differences these physiological states present in the postpartum period. Considering the extent to which the body during birth has been stretched, torn, and potentially cut, the level of postpartum nutrition knowledge in health professionals is underwhelming.

Pregnancy spacing—or more simply, the length of time between pregnancies—is one factor that can impact nutritional status and provides an initial model of just how long the body needs to recover from birth. We know that a close succession of pregnancies and periods of lactation worsen the mother's nutritional status.[3] This is in part because of the time it takes for the body to recover from the physiological stresses of the preceding pregnancy before the stresses of the next pregnancy occur. The current recommendation for pregnancy spacing is 18 months to 2 years due to the impact of the physiological stressors of birth; however, other factors impact maternal nutritional status other than the birth interval.

Maternal nutritional status postpartum is also affected by the initiation and duration of breast-feeding, which varies for each woman. Thus, the picture of just how long it takes women's bodies to recover from the nutritional burden of birth becomes even more unclear. Some literature goes on to attempt to define a recuperative period that includes the time between pregnancies and lactation to determine the nutritional state.[4] However, this data goes to show that simply identifying pregnancy spacing is not a strong enough marker to help us identify just how long the body needs to replenish nutritionally during this postpartum period.

Without clear markers on just how long it takes for women's bodies to nutritionally recover from childbirth, how can we then determine guidelines for adequate nutrition during this period? Below, I will define some of the many variables that can be present during birth and postpartum that may differentiate individual nutritional needs. While the requirements for nutrition during postpartum go beyond the scope of what is listed below, I will narrow in on the acute recovery phase after birth and the first 40 days to provide a basis for nourishing new mothers in the early postpartum phase.

BIRTH CONSIDERATIONS AND NUTRITIONAL NEEDS

Nutritional considerations for mothers postpartum start with the birth story. Throughout pregnancy and certainly during the last trimester, when the uterus has grown to stretch to the size of a watermelon (five times the prepregnancy size!), we know that nutrient needs increase to support a growing fetus and, hormonally, the body is preparing for the marathon of birth. During labor and birth the tissues of the body shift drastically, the uterus contracts and shrinks, and a cascade of hormones set in to prepare for lactation.

Secondary to this are the additional energy requirements of long labors, birth interventions, blood loss, and, potentially, birth injury to the pelvic floor and tissues. All of the above, including preexisting health conditions prior to and during pregnancy, affect recovery time and impact nutritional needs. Some additional factors that affect nutritional requirements postpartum are explored below.

PHYSIOLOGICAL BIRTH

Physiological birth variables that impact nutritional demands include length of labor, intensity of pushing, birth interventions, and any damage to tissues, such as vaginal tearing and episiotomy. A mother who has a longer, more intense labor will require more calorically for repletion. Blood loss during birth can affect maternal postpartum iron status, and tearing and cutting of the perineum impacts tissues that require additional protein and micronutrients.

CESAREAN BIRTH

Variables included in nutritional repletion for cesarean birth include whether the delivery mode was planned or unplanned, as a mother who experiences an emergency cesarean section will likely have already labored and progressed to a certain extent, putting additional stressors on the body and, thus, increasing her energy needs. Additionally, we know that not only is cesarean birth a major abdominal surgery, which raises nutritional requirements for healing, but the risk of blood loss and subsequent maternal anemia is higher in this type of birth as well.

ACUTE RECOVERY

The acute recovery phase begins immediately after birth and typically lasts 7 to 14 days. It is the most nutritionally demanding time postpartum. Immediately after birth, many mothers will experience physical symptoms such as fatigue, soreness, night sweats, and overall depletion as the body physiologically shifts to meeting the energy demands of recovery. During this phase and after delivery of the placenta, a cascade of hormones shift the body from the pregnant state to the non-pregnant state to induce lactation. All of these shifts, on top of the emotional roller coaster that accompanies birth, work to inform the picture of postpartum recovery. Below I cover some of the key hormones at play during the first two weeks after birth to demonstrate just how significant these shifts are on postpartum recovery:

Responsible for the many emotional shifts during the pregnant state (remember crying at the commercials? Yup, you can thank these hormones), *estrogen and progesterone* are at peak levels during pregnancy. Placenta delivery occurs around one to two hours after birth, and estrogen and progesterone levels begin to plummet as the body transitions to promote lactation, whether a woman decides to or is able to breastfeed or not.

- **Endorphins,** which run sky high after the marathon of birth, begin to level off after the first 24 to 48 hours after birth, and many women notice a shift in mood/emotions in response. It takes the body one to two weeks to move back to prepregnancy hormonal levels of estrogen and progesterone. This shift can leave a woman with an ungrounded, unfamiliar feeling now recognized as the *baby blues*. Feelings of irritability, mood swings, and anxiety can run high during this time.

- **Oxytocin,** which helps the uterus contract during birth to deliver the baby, also provides that dose of complete awe and adoration for your baby immediately after birth. Oxytocin is on the rise during the one- to two-week transition period after birth and helps to promote mother-infant bonding and feelings of attachment and attunement. It is important to note the oxytocin feedback loop that is present during breastfeeding, whereby oxytocin is released via the pituitary gland in the brain in response to a baby suckling at the breast, thus promoting a release of oxytocin.

- **Relaxin** is produced at a rate 10 times higher than usual during pregnancy to inhibit premature childbirth. It also assists with softening ligaments and joints (notably the opening and softening of the cervix) to help accommodate the birth of the infant. Relaxin continues to be produced during breastfeeding and affects all of the joints; thus, pain from looser and less stable junctions may continue until after lactation ceases. Even without the continuation of lactation, it takes around five months for relaxin levels to normalize.

PREPARING TO BREASTFEED

Immediately after delivery, whether a mother chooses to breastfeed or not, the body prepares hormonally to breastfeed. The delivery of the placenta triggers a drastic drop in progesterone and increases the hormone *prolactin*, which assists in increasing the volume of milk in the breast (surprising to most women is that milk secretion actually begins in pregnancy!). Should a mother continue to breastfeed, her milk volume increases in response to the infant's demand. The rise of oxytocin triggers the intense thirst experienced by mothers after birth and increases nutritional demand. Just as in pregnancy, when the baby's nutritional needs are prioritized, lactation places high demands on the mother's energy and protein stores and needs to be supported with an increase in overall nutritional intake.

It is important to note that for those women who are either unable to breastfeed or who choose not to, nutritional needs still increase simply due to the overwhelming energy demands of birth and the acute postpartum phase. As discussed, if a woman will not continue to lactate, her body will still move through the physiological process of what is known as lactogenesis (aka making breastmilk) and, thus, mobilizes energy reserves until lactation is discontinued. If a mother is recovering from birth and non-lactating, this is identified as the *recuperative period* when nutrition is still extremely important for maternal repletion.

FORTY DAYS AND BEYOND

After the first two weeks of acute recovery comes the next phase of early postpartum, known as *the first 40 days*. This time frame lasts six to eight weeks and has become a hallmark of sanctioned recovery time around the globe. Physiologically, the body is still in repletion mode, and while energy needs are not as acutely high as they were after birth or during the first week, hunger and appetite are often at peak levels as the body aims to heal.

During this time period, women are adjusting and settling into their new routine with their newborn. Given the erratic sleep schedule that usually ensues, they are frequently exhausted and fatigued. Physiologically, hormones are leveling out as the mother-baby dyad learns breastfeeding, postpartum bleeding (known as *lochia*) continues for four to six weeks, and healing of the pelvic floor and surgical incisions occurs as well. During this time, it is important to place an emphasis on adequate sleep, limiting physically straining and exhaustive tasks, and accessing regular, nutrient-dense meals.

Emotionally, the early postpartum period is filled with transitions and reorientation of the self. This shift into becoming a mother and the complexities that accompany it is known as *matrescence*. As a mother recovers physically and nutritionally from birth, she also experiences a big internal emotional and spiritual shift that requires not just physical nourishment from food, but also nourishment in the form of emotional support from loved ones.

It goes without saying that regardless of how your baby is brought into the world, birth and postpartum are actually more nutritionally demanding times than pregnancy and need to be prioritized in order to optimize your recovery and outcomes. Below, I will dive into how we can nourish and replenish during postpartum, 40 days after birth and beyond.

Chapter 2

Recovery and Energy Needs

Now that you have a better understanding of postpartum recovery time, we can focus on energy needs and the role this plays in healing. Nutrition is emphasized in pregnancy, as it is easier in a sense to comprehend the need for increased nutrition during this time. We now know that postpartum nutrition needs actually increase, even from the pregnant state. While the body is not growing a baby, the process of wound and incision healing, tissue healing, and the beginning of lactogenesis necessitates maximizing nutrition.

In the discussion of nutritional energy needs postpartum, it is important to avoid fixating on prescriptive caloric guidelines. For many women, fixating on caloric intake during pregnancy and postpartum can activate dieting mentality, disordered eating behaviors, or even eating disorder symptoms (more on this later). To remain mindful of this possibility, I use the term "energy" in place of "calories."

Similar to pregnancy, where energy guidelines are provided for each trimester, energy guidelines are provided for postpartum. Energy needs vary from woman to woman and are determined by a variety of factors such as metabolism, muscle mass, metabolic rate, and a history of dieting/disordered eating, to name a few. The generic recommendation to consume additional energy postpartum seems to only apply to mothers who are lactating and leaves out those who are recovering from birth.

We do know that there is an increased need for energy to replenish stores in the acute phase after birth and that these energy needs tend to decrease slightly after this initial two-week period (read: You will be *hungry* after birth). After the acute phase, energy needs remain high, regardless of whether a woman continues to lactate or not; however, continued lactation puts further demands on a woman's body and thus requires more energy intake. Putting a specific number on how much you should eat can not only feel restrictive, but can often lead you to undereat and turn away from the hunger cues your body gives you.

Given that Western cultures live in a diet-centric and weight loss–focused society, the focus on energy needs seems to stem from an emphasis on weight loss, even from the early days of postpartum. It is important to acknowledge how quickly the dialogue seems to shift for mothers after they give birth. Following the hugely taxing process of labor and delivery, from both a physical and emotional stance, mothers deserve infinite admiration for bringing life into the world.

The general dialogue regarding weight loss postpartum is in alignment with the broken pattern we discussed earlier around the six-week expectation of normalcy after birth. Many women are told that after this six-week period they should "get back on track" with the practices they used pre-pregnancy (whether it be restricting foods, exercising vigorously, etc.) in an obligatory effort to "get their body back." Focusing on weight loss postpartum has been shown to lead to higher instances of negative body image, increased risk of perinatal mood and anxiety disorders, and disordered eating/eating disorders.[5] It is important to reframe the expectation for postpartum away from weight loss and to acknowledge that weight variations after birth are going to be diverse and dependent on many different factors. Individual factors affecting weight shifts after birth include prepregnancy weight, hormonal balance, continuation of lactation, and a history of dieting and disordered eating/eating disorders as this severely impacts metabolic rate.

So instead of offering prescriptive, weight- and energy-focused guidelines for postpartum, I offer the following guidelines for meeting your energy needs postpartum:

- **Focus on becoming attuned with your hunger and fullness cues to guide energy needs postpartum.** Our bodies have infinite wisdom and complex hormonal and metabolic processes that assist us in regulating our intake. Expect to experience an increase in hunger postpartum without putting judgement or a timeline on it. Many women struggle with honoring that they will likely have larger appetites. This increase should be expected as the body recovers, and just how long this continues depends on the many variables discussed above.

- **Maximize nutrients and repletion rather than focusing on foods to avoid or minimize.** Postpartum should be a time of healing and repletion for the body physically and emotionally. Emphasis should be put on incorporating nutrient-dense foods that provide sustenance. Avoiding or eliminating food groups (dieting), and trying to minimize or suppress hunger/appetite take away from the body's attempt to heal and repair and impact overall nutritional status.

- **Adopt an all-foods-fit and flexible eating style.** Embracing an all-foods-fit mentality pairs well with postpartum. All foods fit means that while certain foods have the capacity to boost nutrition and promote healing, no one food has the power to heal or hurt postpartum. Nutrition is synergistic, meaning it is a combination of different foods that promotes optimal health and well-being over time. Adopting a mindset of flexibility serves well in the shift to motherhood, as your ability to prepare and tend to meals is different from life before baby.

- **Incorporate body respect as a practice.** Body respect involves acknowledging pregnancy and birth without a focus on weight, shape, or size. It also involves making space for nourishment postpartum out of respect for our bodies' need to rest and heal versus fixing/controlling.

NOURISHING TRADITIONS

You may be wondering if there are specific foods or a diet that will support postpartum. Currently, Westernized culture does not have any standard postpartum practice relative to specific foods. Thus, I sought to gather the common themes emphasized by other cultures to see how closely they align with nutrition science and how we can apply these practices for postpartum.

Common in ancient medical principles is the emphasis on food and specific food properties in healing. During postpartum, a recurring theme is that mothers should consume certain foods to promote health restoration and avoid certain foods thought to promote illness. Mothers are viewed as vulnerable physically after birth. This duality with food (known as yin and yang) can be seen in Ayurvedic medicine and traditional Chinese medicine, where certain foods are categorized by intrinsic hot categories (hot food), thought to significantly raise the body's heat, or cold categories (cold food), thought to reduce the body's heat. Balancing these foods is thought to help rid the postpartum body of excess blood to bring healing. Many cultures view the pregnant state as *hot* due to the presence of extra blood volume, and postpartum is seen as *cold* as there is blood loss after birth.[6]

Though the types of foods vary depending on what is local and familiar to the region (spicy soup in Mexico, hot curry in India), the principles regarding different nutritional practices in many cultures have familiar themes. Some of the interconnected postpartum nutritional principles around the globe are:

- **Warming and well-seasoned foods.** Many cultures emphasize warmth in foods. This refers both to temperature (largely related to the belief regarding hot/cold properties) and also to warmth from spices added to dishes during cooking. Broths, teas, soups, and stews all fit the bill, the warmth providing both comfort and additional fluids that are lost during birth. In Westernized cultures, women are commonly steered away from spicy foods postpartum if they are breastfeeding, as it is thought that this spice will lead to intolerance in the infant. In fact, this is inaccurate. Furthermore, spice is encouraged regardless of whether a mother is breastfeeding or not. Spices are rich in antioxidants and essential oils and add flavor and warmth to meals.

- **High-fat and -protein foods to support tissue repair, support breastmilk production, and build up blood stores.** High-fat foods in the postpartum diet provide substantial energy, add flavor, and aid in the absorption of certain vitamins. High-protein options such as animal foods supplement iron stores and help build up blood that may have been lost through delivery.

- **Carbohydrates, starches, and vegetables that are cooked versus raw.** Cooked and warm grains, starches, and vegetables are thought to aid in digestion by providing fiber and micronutrients. Many cultures believe that when foods are cooked, the body can extract the energy and nutrients without as much energy. During pregnancy, the digestive system handles an enormous amount of pressure from the growing uterus. Many mothers express feeling as if their digestive system is sluggish postpartum, for good reason!

The purpose of highlighting some of the common practices in other cultures is to be able to derive wisdom from these rituals and marry them with evidence-based nutritional science and, of course, practicality. Many of the above principles seem intuitive—a warm, nourishing bowl of stew after birth sounds like just what the body needs. However, it is important to emphasize the need for consuming varied foods from the different macronutrients in a way that is practical and functional for modern-day life. In the section to follow, I will cover how this does not always look like slow-cooked meals that include exotic spices and ingredients.

The recipes found in this cookbook infuse traditional practices as listed above while integrating the basics of adequate nutrition for postpartum recovery in modern-day motherhood.

BASIC MACRONUTRIENTS FOR POSTPARTUM RECOVERY

While we discussed some of the important principles to keep in mind to meet energy needs, it can be helpful to focus on what to put together to build nutrient-dense meals and snacks. Macronutrients are the building blocks of the energy we consume and come in three forms: carbohydrates, protein, and dietary fat. Each macronutrient plays a specific role in the body, and most foods contain a mix of all of these macronutrients. This section introduces how to support postpartum recovery by providing appropriate combinations of these nutrients in the diet.

Food works synergistically in the body; thus, combining the macronutrients works best to support nutrition. When we eat specific macronutrients, they are broken down through digestion and provide cells with energy. Which macronutrients we consume and in what quantities influences blood sugar levels, which impact physical energy levels, mood, hormonal balance, and overall health. When we eat one macronutrient in isolation, it impacts the body by causing a spike in blood sugar level, which can lead to negative physical symptoms such as irritability, fatigue, and, of course, hunger.

For example, consuming a carbohydrate such as crackers in isolation will increase the blood sugar level quickly but after a short time will cause the blood sugar level to drop (bring on the hanger!). Pairing those crackers with either peanut butter or cheese (which contain both protein and dietary fat) provides a combination of macronutrients and thus delivers a stable blood sugar level for a longer period of time, which = a happy mom.

RULE OF THREE

The "rule" in "rule of three" doesn't mean a rigid guideline to follow. Rather it's a gentle guideline that can help steer moms toward feeling their best physically after birth (no mom has time to feel increasingly irritable, hungry, or fatigued!). Pairing the macronutrients together at meals and snacks can help provide the stable blood sugar that promotes sustained energy and mood through the day.

The rule of three entails including all three macronutrients in some form to provide stabilized energy at meals. Most meals that come to mind naturally involve this combination; however, in our diet culture, which often encourages skimping on certain foods, we must be mindfully aware to include these nutrients at meals.

Most nutritional information contains specific reference ranges, recommended grams, etc. Reference ranges provide markers for certain nutrients, such as the Recommended Daily Allowance (RDA), which outlines the average level of intake of nutrients needed for 97 to 98 percent of individuals, and the Daily Reference Intake (DRI), which gives the general reference range of nutrient intake, varying by age, life cycle, and sex. These references provide general information about the needs of women who continue lactation; however, they lack guidelines around postpartum mothers who are healing and do not continue lactation.

While this information can be inherently valuable, in practice I have found the needs of women so variable that I cannot emphasize the benefit of individualized nutrition counseling enough. The information below highlights the function and need for these nutrients in the diet and I intentionally leave out ranges.

Overall, individuals who consume a variety of foods in moderation in accordance with their hunger/fullness will be able to meet their nutritional needs through "foods-first" approach (without the use of supplements). Depending on the individual's unique health history, lifestyle, and dietary intake, specific nutrition interventions and recommendations may be needed around the intake of nutrients. I recommend working with a skilled nutrition therapist for individualized recommendations.

If you are interested in accessing more specifics on these ranges outside of consultation with a registered dietitian, you can find the complete list of Dietary Reference Intakes (DRIs) for macronutrients and total water at the National Institutes of Health website, Office of Dietary Supplements.

CARBOHYDRATES

Carbohydrates are perhaps the best-known macronutrient and easily one of the most controversial. Carbohydrates have the most impact on our blood sugar levels, as the breakdown of carbohydrates provides the body's preferred source of fuel: glucose.

Carbohydrate is broken down in the body and the glucose that results fuels the brain and body. The primary functions of carbohydrates are to provide energy, regulate blood sugar levels, protect muscle mass (by sparing use of protein), and aid in promoting digestion. Carbohydrates also provide a release of serotonin, a neurotransmitter that promotes feelings of well-being and, in motherhood, can promote maternal behavior.[7] Just how much an individual needs to consume carbohydrates is individualized based on health history and need. However, in postpartum the general guideline is to ensure that at least 50 to 60 percent of your meal is composed of carbohydrates.

Often when discussing carbohydrates, "good" and "bad" come into play. While I steer away from using these labels in an all-foods-fit mentality, I can bring attention to differences between complex and simple carbohydrates, which refer to the carbohydrates structure.

Complex carbohydrates are composed of starches and fiber such as whole grains, beans, and fruits and vegetables, while *simple carbohydrates* are often naturally occurring in milk and other foods such as sugars and fruit juice. Complex carbohydrate are supportive in postpartum as these foods contain a higher content of fiber, which provides support for digestion and blood sugar balance. To practice the principles of moderation, variety, and balance, include both of these types of carbohydrates in accordance with individual needs and preferences.

Foods that provide primarily carbohydrates include starches such as bread, rice, pasta, quinoa, legumes, potatoes, and starchy vegetables. Fruits and dairy also provide carbohydrates.

PROTEIN

Protein during postpartum recovery is essential. Protein's primary functions include serving as a major building block for muscle and tissue, aiding immune function, and helping to provide satiety by delaying gastric emptying. There is a total of 20 different amino acids, which, when compiled together, form a protein.

Some of these amino acids are termed nonessential because the body makes them, and the others are termed essential amino acids because they must be consumed through food sources as the body cannot produce these. Many proteins are building blocks for hormones and assist with transporting vitamins and minerals via circulation. During labor, birth, and lactation, the protein stores that were built up during pregnancy to support the growing fetus are mobilized for repair work.

Protein needs postpartum increase to support healing of any birth injuries to muscles or tissues, such as in the case of perineal tearing, an episiotomy, or a cesarean birth. Vegetarian and vegan diets both come up in conversations around postnatal nutrition, often in relation to protein. These dietary patterns were previously thought to pose a nutritional risk, and while they do necessitate careful planning, research has shown that these can be appropriate for the postpartum period.[8]

Food sources that provide protein include animal foods such as beef and poultry, seafood, dairy products, and eggs. Vegetarian sources include beans and legumes, tofu, edamame, meat alternatives, nuts, and seeds.

DIETARY FAT

Dietary fat is a critical nutrient throughout life. Dietary fats are essential for protecting vital organs, enhancing absorption of fat-soluble vitamins such as vitamin A, D, E, and K, and brain growth and development. During pregnancy, fat assists largely with fetal brain development as well as cell and skin formation. In postpartum, fat is essential to provide long-lasting energy, increase satiety at meals, enhance the taste and texture of food, and protect mental health by acting on neurotransmitters and hormones. Fat promotes the release of appetite hormones that promote satisfaction and satiety (two things moms need during quick meals!).

Many know the rigid categorization of "good" and "bad" dietary fats; however, an all-foods-fit approach emphasizes that including a variety of all fats is essential to meet nutritional needs.

The two major fat groups are unsaturated and saturated fats. These names refer to their chemical makeup. Unsaturated fats consist of monounsaturated and polyunsaturated fats, and the United States Department of Agriculture (USDA) recommends that individuals focus on sourcing fats from these sources as higher intakes of unsaturated fats is linked to lower incidences of cardiovascular disease.[9] Common sources of unsaturated fats are found primarily in plant foods such as oils, nuts and seeds, and cold-water fish.

Saturated fats, thought to be "bad," are also important to include in the variety of fats consumed. Many foods that contain saturated fat also contain cholesterol, which is a critical building block of cell membranes and a precursor to making vitamin D and certain hormones. Saturated fats are often found in animal foods, which are rich in other micronutrients valuable for healing during the postpartum period. Common food sources of saturated fat include meat and poultry, eggs, butter, cheese, and palm/coconut oils.

Noteworthy for postpartum moms are omega-3 and omega-6 fatty acids, which are types of unsaturated fats. Omega-3 fatty acids have been given the most attention in recent years for the significant role they play in fetal brain functioning and development. There are three main types of omega-3 fatty acids: alpha-linoleic acid (ALA), eicosapentaenoic acid (EPA), and docosahexae-noic acid (DHA). Growing evidence also shows that these fatty acids can have a positive impact on preventing and treating perinatal mood disorders.[10] Major sources of omega-3s are seafood, DHA-fortified products, microalgae supplements, vegetable oils, soybeans, and nuts and seeds. Ensuring that the postpartum diet is rich in a variety of these fats will assist with optimal functioning, provide sustained energy, and promote optimal mood.

FLUIDS

Hydration is a no-brainer during postpartum; almost every new mom will emphasize just how thirsty she is after birth and while breastfeeding! The fluid demands of birth increase the need for repletion in the acute recovery stage as there are fluid losses that accumulate from the intensity and duration of labor, fluids shifts from medications, if administered, and the onset of lactogenesis.

Oxytocin, produced from the initial latch of an infant at the breast, triggers increased thirst, and meeting fluid needs throughout postpartum and lactation is essential to healing tissues, promoting digestion, and preventing hemorrhoids and postpartum swelling. The general recommendation during pregnancy is 10 cups (~2.3 liters) of fluid a day and during lactation is 13 cups (~3.8 liters) of fluid a day. For non-lactating mothers postpartum, I would aim for an intake within the range of 10 to 13 cups daily.[11] Of course, as with nutrition, fluid needs vary depending on an individual's overall health, environment, and overall exertion (this includes exercise, which should be limited during acute postpartum recovery).

MICRONUTRIENTS

Micronutrients consist of vitamins and minerals the body needs to maintain physiological function and provide a myriad of different functions in the body. The all-foods-fit philosophy focuses on consuming a variety of foods that encompass a spectrum of vitamins and minerals. I highlight the micronutrients beneficial during postpartum below, as there are often gaps in the intake of these vitamins and minerals. No need to count micrograms here or be frantic about checking labels. Instead, aim to consume a variety of foods that are rich in colors and texture. Stay in tune with your body's hunger and fullness cues to meet the majority of your micronutrient needs.

As described previously, the Recommended Daily Allowances (RDA) are cited for lactation. However, no reference ranges are given for women who are postpartum and non-lactating. It is a critical gap as we cannot assume that the same nutrient recommendations of prepregnancy levels resume after giving birth. Consult with a registered dietitian for further information regarding specific micronutrient needs based on individual health history and birth experience.

It is recommended to continue to take a prenatal vitamin postpartum for at least six months if you are not breastfeeding or to take you throughout the duration of breastfeeding. Keep in mind that just as during pregnancy, a prenatal vitamin during postpartum should act as an "insurance policy" for filling nutrient gaps, not as a way to meet these needs. The focus should continue to be on consuming real food in moderation, variety, and balance.

IRON

Iron is essential for heme synthesis in the body, which forms hemoglobin and assists with transferring oxygen from the lungs to all tissues. During pregnancy, as blood volume increases, the recommended intake is ~27 mg/day. The recommendation drops to 9 mg/day for lactating women.

This recommendation has been controversial, as even the recommendation for prepregnancy iron intake is higher, at 18 mg/day. This gap is thought to be related to the period of lactational amenorrhea (the absence of menses during lactation); however, this period of amenorrhea varies for each woman depending on the initiation of breastfeeding, exclusivity of breastfeeding (full or partial feeding), and frequency of feedings.

Furthermore, this lower recommendation of iron does not consider the factors during birth and postpartum that may affect iron status postpartum. These include preexisting anemia prenatally, blood loss during or after delivery, and lochia (bloody discharge after birth). Thus, ensuring adequate iron after birth is critical to replenishing stores, particularly in the case of the abovementioned factors.

Both heme and non-heme sources of iron affect the absorption of the mineral in the body. Heme sources of iron are found in animal foods such as meat (especially red meat), poultry, seafood, and fish. Non-heme sources of iron are found in plant foods such as whole grains, nuts, seeds, and legumes. These are less readily absorbable due to the presence of phytates, which inhibit absorption.

To assist with iron absorption of non-heme iron foods, consume iron-rich foods with a source of vitamin C such as citrus fruit or tomatoes, cook foods in a cast-iron skillet, and avoid consumption of calcium-rich foods alongside iron-rich items, as these minerals compete for absorption.

Ensuring adequate intake of iron-rich foods has also shown to help prevent postpartum depression and the common symptoms of iron deficiency such as fatigue, shortness of breath, and difficulty concentrating, all unwelcome symptoms to a sleep-deprived new mom.[12]

VITAMIN D

While the nutrient requirements identified for vitamin D remain stable for prepregnancy and lactation (600 IU), vitamin D deficiency in pregnant women is common. Vitamin D's role as a fat-soluble vitamin means that its concentrations in the body are dependent on diet quality. Ensuring adequate intake postpartum is a concern for women who may have been deficient during pregnancy due to risk factors such as geographical location, darker skin pigmentation, and limited sun exposure.

Maintaining adequate levels of vitamin D is critical for women who are breastfeeding, as maternal vitamin D status influences the concentrations in breastmilk. Currently, the American Academy of Pediatrics recommends supplementing exclusively breastfed infants with 400 IU vitamin D serum as the factors affecting maternal vitamin D status are variable. Some recent studies have shown that supporting maternal intake of adequate vitamin D can promote optimal serum vitamin D levels in breastmilk; however, it is unclear how much vitamin D new moms should supplement with.[13] Therefore, including vitamin D-rich foods such as egg yolks, fish such as salmon, tuna, and mackerel, cheese, mushrooms, fortified milks, and cereals in your diet can support adequate levels of vitamin D in the body.

VITAMIN A

Vitamin A requirements increase to 1,300 mcg during lactation. Again, we do not have data to provide a marker for this vitamin in women who are postpartum and not lactating. But this nutrient's vital functions in immunity, cell growth, and the maintenance of organs are critical for all women postpartum. Two forms of vitamin A are available through foods: preformed vitamin A (retinol), which is found in liver, fish oil, milk, and eggs, and provitamin A (carotenoids), found in orange and yellow fruits and vegetables such as sweet potatoes, peppers, tomatoes, and cantaloupe as well as dark, leafy greens.

B VITAMINS

The B vitamins include eight different types of vitamins (also called the B vitamin complex), each of which serves an individual function. The complex assists in the formation of blood cells, tissue production, and metabolizing food into energy. The nutrient requirements for B vitamins increase in both pregnancy and lactation. Vitamin B12 is found only in animal products and some fortified, plant-based products. Vitamin B12 deficiency can lead to neurological symptoms and anemia. Good sources of vitamin B12 include beef, pork, poultry, dairy products, and eggs.

IODINE

Recommended intake for iodine increases in pregnancy and lactation (220 mcg and 290 mcg, respectively). Iodine plays a role in immunity, metabolism, and thyroid function. Thyroid hormones regulate many metabolic reactions in the body and are required for infant nervous system development. Sources of iodine to include are eggs, fish, shellfish, pork, iodized salt, and seaweed (one of the most iodine-rich sources, albeit an uncommon item in most diets).

ZINC

Zinc promotes cell growth, maintains immunity, and supports normal growth and development through the life stages. As zinc requirements increase during pregnancy and lactation, highlighting nutrient sources of zinc can support adequate consumption. Oysters, red meat, poultry, beans, and nuts all provide a dose of this essential mineral. As with iron, phytates present in foods such as whole grains and legumes may inhibit absorption of zinc; thus, animal sources of zinc are more bioavailable.

CHOLINE

Choline serves as a metabolite for the formation of cell membranes in the body in addition to serving critical brain and nervous system functions. Even though choline needs are at an all-time high during pregnancy and lactation (450 mg and 550 mg, respectively), most women are not meeting these intake ranges. Many prenatal vitamins do not contain choline, so consuming choline-rich foods can mend this gap. Foods rich in choline are meat, poultry, eggs, nuts, milk, fish, beans, and some cruciferous vegetables such as broccoli, brussels sprouts, and cauliflower.

Chapter 3

Lactation

We can't have a discussion around postnatal nutrition without including the nutritional needs that support lactation. In Western culture, we are finally catching up to other countries that have long held breastfeeding in high regard and cultivated networks of support to assist mothers in continuing breastfeeding.

Breastfeeding is natural for mothers (however, that does not mean it is easy!), as nature designed it. It provides countless health benefits for both mothers and their babies. It seems we learn more and more each day about how valuable breastfeeding can be in brain and growth development and decreasing risk of infections for both mother and baby (no wonder it is termed "liquid gold"). As a board-certified lactation consultant (what is considered the gold standard in the lactation profession, being certified by the International Board of Lactation Consultant Examiners) and registered dietitian, I have interest not only in supporting mothers in learning the dance of breastfeeding with their baby but also ensuring that this nutritionally taxing period of lactation is supported with adequate nutrition.

During pregnancy, the body stored up energy to ensure that your baby would be supported nutritionally after birth. In lactation, these energy stores are then mobilized to produce milk for your little one each time they breastfeed. Energy needs during breastfeeding are a common discussion topic. The Institute of Medicine (IOM) has estimated that breastfeeding women utilize ~500 additional calories a day. This varies based on individual metabolic rate, birth experience, single or multiple birth, and the frequency of feedings (which determine how much milk your body produces in response). Again, no need to count calories here, as tuning into hunger and fullness will allow you to satisfy the increase in macronutrients your body needs. Intensity of hunger during breastfeeding varies by individual; some women experience a marked increase in appetite that does not seem to subside and others notice peaks of increased hunger after breastfeeding sessions.

One barrier to breastfeeding for many women is feeling as if their diet needs to be perfect in order to breastfeed. Given that one of the biggest challenges postpartum is finding time for food preparation, cooking, and shopping to meet these needs, it is easy to see how this can set women up with unrealistic expectations. In fact, there is no special diet required to breastfeed. Milk is made from the blood, and what a mother intakes via her diet is all that is needed to produce milk. While studying the composition of breastmilk over time, research has shown that even moderately malnourished women produce adequate breastmilk.[14] Of course, while it is encouraging to know how adaptable the body is at providing adequate nutrition for infants, it does come at a "nutritional cost" for the mother. Without adequate body stores of energy or essential vitamins and minerals, the body will draw on nutritional reserves (many of which were mobilized during birth and the acute phase of postpartum) and can become depleted.

While there is no special diet for breastfeeding mothers, nutrition requirements do increase during this time. Again, tuning into hunger and fullness typically satisfies your body's macronutrient and micronutrient needs. Exceptions to this are women who are undernourished or on a restricted diet such as those on vegetarian or vegan diets, those with a history of gastric bypass surgery, or those who have malabsorptive disorders. In these situations, vitamin and mineral supplementation and careful planning with a registered dietitian is warranted to prevent deficiencies in the breastmilk. Outside of these specific scenarios, some tips for meeting nutrition requirements during breastfeeding are below:

- Eat in accordance with hunger and fullness and drink to thirst, keeping snacks and a water bottle next to your during nursing sessions.
- Consume caffeine in moderation; each baby's tolerance will vary.
- If consuming a vegetarian or vegan diet, ensure a well-planned diet with adequate B vitamins (specifically B12, found in animal products), protein, and iron.
- Keep energy levels high throughout the day by consuming nutrient-dense meals and snacks every two to three hours.
- Check with your physician on the medications and herbs you take during breastfeeding.

While some variations of normal exist, breastfeeding mothers can consume a normal diet and enjoy foods in moderation, variety, and balance to meet nutritional needs. When you introduce a variety of foods into the maternal diet, you set the stage to expose diverse flavors and tastes to your infant later on during the introduction of solid foods. A common concern in regard to nutrition and breastfeeding is the belief that you need to avoid certain foods when an infant becomes fussy or experiences gas pains. While no parent is immune to an infant who experiences these bouts of discomfort, research shows that only about 5 percent of infants react to something in the maternal diet.[15] However, many cultures have similar beliefs about breastfeeding, and mothers are dissuaded from consuming spicy foods, cruciferous vegetables, or even cold liquids, thought to contribute to fussiness and colic in an infant. To this, I emphasize that breastmilk is made from the blood, not the contents of the stomach, and thus, the incidences when an infant reacts to something in a mother's diet are low.

While it is the exception to the rule, the signs of a hypersensitivity in an infant that is directly related to what the mom eats can include skin concerns such as dry skin, rash, or eczema; gastrointestinal problems such as diarrhea, vomiting, or bloody stools; and overall fussiness such as difficulty falling or staying asleep and irritability. Eliminating a suspected food item for a day or two may bring relief; however, it typically takes two to three weeks to fully eliminate a trigger from the mother's body (as in the case of a reaction of cow's milk protein).

To conclude, I want to emphasize that the decision to breastfeed is seldom based only on the knowledge of just how valuable it is nutritionally for both mother and baby. Rather, a mother's physical and emotional ability to do so and her access to skilled breastfeeding support also come into play. Just as with information around nutrition, discussions around breastfeeding can be charged, and I want to acknowledge that while breastfeeding is the norm, there are many women who, after informed consent, choose not to breastfeed their baby or are unable to for a variety of reasons. For this group of mothers, I cannot emphasize enough that the discussions regarding nutrition in this book are still just as relevant to you for nutritional healing!

You are more than your breastmilk. A variety of emotions can be present postpartum simply due to the physiological state, and facing barriers to breastfeeding or experiencing challenges in your journey can come with feelings of anger, frustration, and grief. Acknowledging that your decision is what is best for you, your baby, and your family, discussing your decision with your care team, and ensuring that you have access to skilled support such as a lactation consultant or a perinatal therapist can hold space for you during this process.

Chapter 4

Mental Health

With any huge life transition, there is room for a range of emotions, from joy and elation to anger, grief, and loss. The journey of motherhood is certainly filled with vulnerability as you learn a new role, experience changes physically and physiologically, and navigate new relationship dynamics. In the midst of these changes, postpartum blues, also known as "the baby blues," is common after birth to up to two to three weeks thereafter. More than 50 percent of new mothers experience this shift in mood. Some studies suggest this number is actually close to even 80 percent.

Common experiences during the baby blues include tearfulness, increased stress and anxiety, and difficulties with sleep or appetite unrelated to newborn care. These changes are within the realm of normal after birth as hormones shift, fatigue sets in, and the tasks of caring for a newborn come into play. During this time, partners and families can support women by providing support with newborn care, supporting basic needs such as meals, allowing time for rest and hygiene, and providing plenty of affirmation and reassurance.

For many women, this time of baby blues comes and goes; however, for others, symptoms intensify and can become more severe. Postpartum depression (PPD) is estimated to occur in 15 to 20 percent of new mothers and is defined as occurring after four weeks to one year postpartum. Some research suggests that the onset can be even later, and while we are continuing to discover more and more about the different factors that impact risk for women, there is still much to learn. We do know that symptoms of PPD include sadness, decreased interest in activities (anhedonia), difficulty focusing, anger and irritability, changes in appetite, and withdrawal. Risk factors for developing PPD include a prior history of depression/mental health concerns, significant life stressors, and a lack of support during the postpartum period. A relationship has also been shown between breastfeeding difficulties and cultural factors that may impact a woman's risk of developing PPD.

Postpartum anxiety (PPA) often overlaps with postpartum depression (PPD) during the postpartum period. It is common to have some of the symptoms of PPA overlap with PPD and for women to experience excessive worry, fear, difficulty concentrating, or having a constant sense of dread. It is important to note that the symptoms listed above for both PPD and PPA are not "one size fits all." An individual may have some but not all of the symptoms, and these states do vacillate. However, they typically last longer than two weeks and impact a sense of well-being and functioning.

With both PPD and PPA, alongside other perinatal mood and anxiety disorders, nutrition can play a crucial role in prevention and reduction of severity. Some general recommendations to support optimal mental health are listed below:

- Maintain a well-balanced diet using the framework provided in Chapter 2. Include adequate amounts of all macronutrients and nutrients that can be related to mood disorders. Nutrients of concern include iron, vitamin B12, vitamin D, and omega-3 fatty acids (DHA). Work with a registered dietitian to review current intake and supplementation needs, if indicated.

- Navigate changes in appetite by adjusting meal timing appropriately. It is important to note that appetite can shift in both directions, increasing or decreasing. Implementing small, frequent meals, setting meal reminders, and eating meals with family can provide support.

- Focus on stabilizing blood sugar levels. Blood sugar swings can affect mood stability, so work to implement the rule of threes discussed in Chapter 2 to ensure balanced blood sugar after meals.

- Be mindful of caffeine and alcohol intake. In some individuals, caffeine intake can activate anxious thoughts/feelings. Alcohol is a neurotoxin and a depressant, and can intensify mood-related symptoms.

- Engage in mindful movement. Movement may be challenging but is an important component in mental health for its relationship to increasing serotonin and dopamine (feel-good neuro-chemicals) and endorphins. Start small and acknowledge that your body is still physically healing. Gentle stretching and yoga are great places to start (also, get adequate vitamin D from the sun!).

- Get adequate sleep. Life with a newborn shifts normal sleep schedules. If you are struggling with a perinatal mood or anxiety disorder, finding support to get adequate sleep is essential. To start, ask for support from others to care for the baby and minimize blue light from technology before bed, as this can disrupt melatonin, and identify consistent sleep and wake times.

- Connect with a therapist who specializes in perinatal health. This is essential to provide psychotherapy and individualized support and resources for connecting with other new mothers.

- Speak with your providers (midwife, OBGYN, therapist, lactation consultant) about a referral for a medication assessment as needed. They can assist with determining if pharmacological support is warranted and would be supportive.

Chapter 5

Dieting Postpartum

Almost all women are subjected to sociocultural pressure during the postpartum period and experience a level of dissatisfaction with their body after birth. This pressure from widespread cultural ideals and the media can exacerbate mental health concerns and put women at risk for disordered eating practices, increased body dissatisfaction, and, if breastfeeding, decreased self-efficacy.[16]

Navigating life with a newborn brings on changes in every arena—physically, emotionally, and spiritually—and many women can experience shifts in their identity and feel ungrounded. Oftentimes, sitting with this discomfort physically and emotionally can translate to projecting this discomfort onto the body with thoughts of weight loss/changing. The thought of weight loss can bring up feelings of familiarity (familiarity of life before baby) and the persistent desire to "return to normal." Dieting or disordered eating behavior in a sense provides a familiar feeling and perceived control over circumstances that are profoundly unfamiliar and new.

While these thoughts are understandable in the shifts of early motherhood, dieting and disordered eating are harmful at any period in time, especially during the postpartum period when women are increasingly more vulnerable. Some practices to support these changes during this time are below:

- Understand the true relationship between dieting and disordered eating, and challenge the idea of what you hope they will bring. Over time, these practices actually lower metabolic rate and can cause more weight gain, less physical attunement, and increased body dissatisfaction.
- Practice self-compassion and self-validation (acting and speaking kindly to yourself). Your body has just experienced rapid changes that are unprecedented at any other time of the life cycle. Research proves that practicing self-compassion can decrease concerns around weight/shape.[17]

- Assess your level of attention to media and diet culture that profit off of dieting and weight loss. Curate media consumption that is inclusive of real postpartum experiences and can validate the normalcy of the postpartum body. Find professional and social support from a perinatal or nutrition therapist if you find that body image thoughts are creating constant stress, worry, and preoccupation.

- Connect with other mothers experiencing these shifts for social support. There can be so much healing that can happen just by finding that others are navigating these thoughts alongside you.

POSTPARTUM TIPS AND TOOLS

By now, I have hopefully shed light on just how complex the postnatal period can be and just how vital replenishing nutrition is. Now, some tips to apply all of the knowledge I've introduced and how to use *The Postnatal Cookbook* to support your journey physically, emotionally, and spiritually.

- Plan for postpartum before it occurs! We plan and prepare for the baby; however, we often lack the planning and preparation needed to create space and time after birth. Just as many women create a birth plan, you can work alongside your partner, midwife, or doula to create a plan for postpartum. This can include identifying logistical tasks, delegating home chores, and finding care for other children.

- Ensure that you have resources for support ready and available, even if you end up not needing them. This includes referrals and contact information for trusted professionals such as a lactation consultant, postpartum doula, registered dietitian, and other community resources (mothers' groups, parenting classes, etc.).

- Find support for planning and preparing meals. Use resources such as online shopping and delivery, batch cooking, and prepared ingredients and pantry staples to have on hand. Allow space for meal delivery for nights when cooking feels overwhelming. You can tab the recipes in this book for your partner or family and friends who would like to know how they can help.

The recipes in this book have been prepared to support nutritional healing and promote satisfaction through variety, moderation, and balance! Remember that nutrition is just one of the many factors that make up the landscape of our health. Taking time out to prepare for this season is essential to soaking up all of the beauty and chaos that make up the postnatal period. I hope that the tools in this book will help support you and your family as you navigate this new season of life so you can be fully present, attuned, and nourished throughout!

Chapter 6

Breakfast

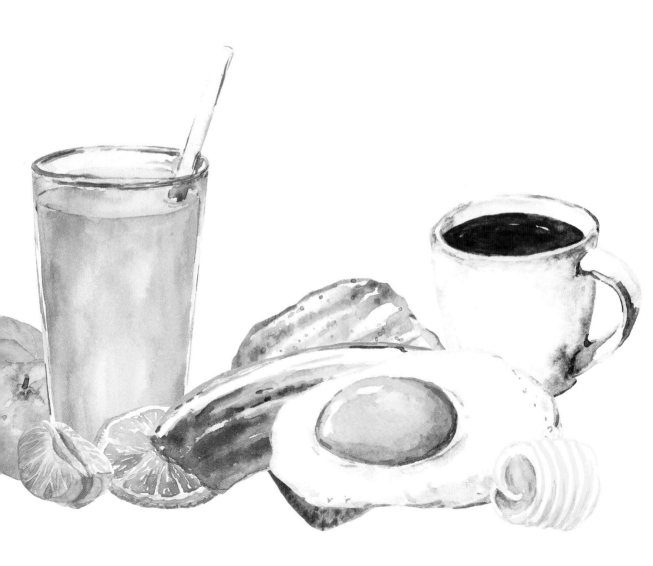

Lemon Raspberry Ricotta Pancakes

Delicious hotcakes get a nutritional boost from Italian ricotta cheese and are packed with bright flavors of lemon and raspberry in this recipe. The ricotta actually makes for the ultimate fluffy pancake as it adds extra moisture to the batter in addition to calcium and protein.

Serves: 6 to 8 | Prep time: 10 minutes | Cook time: 10 minutes

DRY INGREDIENTS

1¼ cups white flour

1 tablespoon baking powder

2 tablespoons granulated sugar

¼ teaspoon salt

WET INGREDIENTS

1 cup full-fat ricotta cheese

juice of 1 lemon

2 eggs

1 cup milk of choice

1 teaspoon vanilla extract

1 tablespoon salted butter, plus more if needed for the griddle

1 (6-ounce) container raspberries

powdered sugar, for dusting

maple syrup, to top

fresh lemon juice, to top

1. In a medium mixing bowl, combine the dry ingredients.

2. In a separate medium mixing bowl, combine the wet ingredients and whisk together until all of the ingredients are smooth and combined.

3. Pour the wet ingredients into the bowl with the dry ingredients and use a spatula to gently fold wet the ingredients into the dry ingredients.

4. Once the mixture is thoroughly combined (with few to no lumps) heat a griddle over medium heat and 1 tablespoon butter on the pan.

5. Using a ¼-cup measuring tool, scoop the batter onto the griddle 2 to 3 at a time. Once bubbles form, use a spatula to check underneath to ensure that it is golden-brown, and flip the pancake to heat the other side, about 2 to 3 minutes.

6. Allow the other side to cook until golden-brown and remove from the griddle. Repeat this process until all of the batter has been used.

7. When preparing to serve, muddle the raspberries to top the pancakes by using a fork to press the berries and create a jam-like texture.

8. Top the pancakes with the raspberries, a dusting of powdered sugar, maple syrup. and fresh lemon juice, as desired.

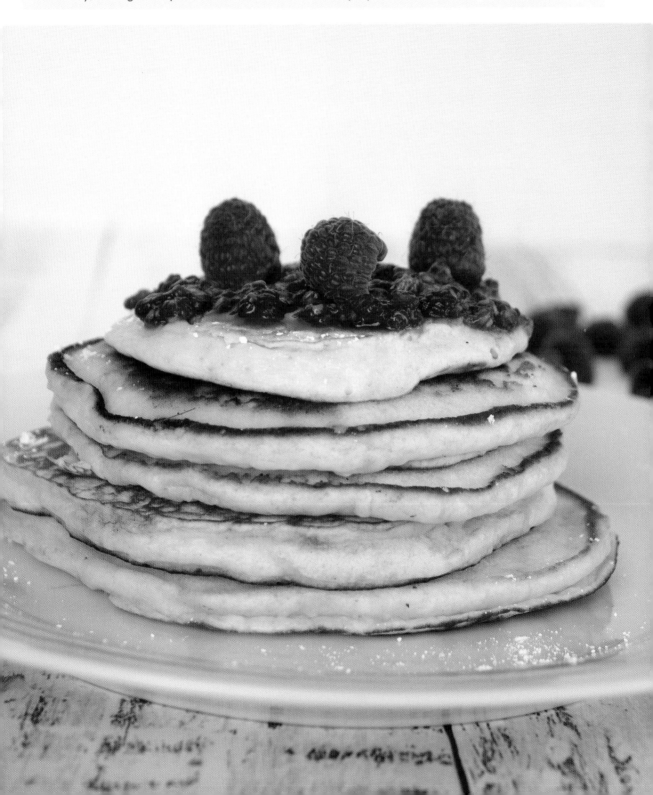

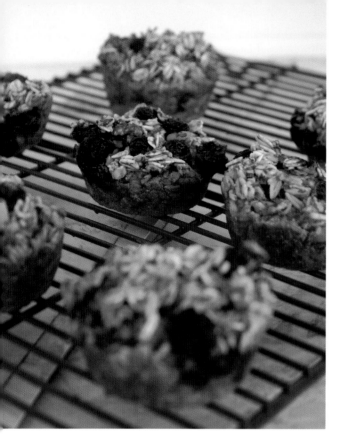

Blueberry Walnut Muffins

Blueberries, oats, and walnuts come together to provide a muffin that is rich in antioxidants, omega-3 fatty acids, iron, and fiber.

Serves: 12 | Prep time: 10 minutes | Cook time: 20 minutes

DRY INGREDIENTS

4 cups old-fashioned oats

1 teaspoon ground cinnamon

1 teaspoon nutmeg

½ teaspoon salt

4 tablespoons ground flaxseeds

2 tablespoons chia seeds

1 cup blueberries, fresh or frozen

½ cup crushed walnuts

WET INGREDIENTS

2⅓ cups milk of choice

¼ cup maple syrup

2 eggs

1 teaspoon vanilla extract

1. Preheat the oven to 375°F.

2. In a large bowl, combine the dry ingredients.

3. In a separate medium bowl, whisk together the milk, syrup, eggs, and vanilla.

4. Combine the wet ingredients with the dry ingredients and stir to fully combine.

5. Grease a muffin pan. Use a ¼-cup measuring scoop to fill the tin.

6. Place the muffin pan in the oven for 20 minutes until, the center of the muffins is set.

#MomHack: Muffins are a perfect one-hand bite. These muffins in particular pack in all the macros you need at once to provide steady energy (carbohydrates, protein, and fat). Like most muffins, these freeze well. Oatmeal muffins will keep in the fridge for five days or can be frozen and stored for three months. Be sure to wrap them individually and you can grab them straight from the freezer to warm them up.

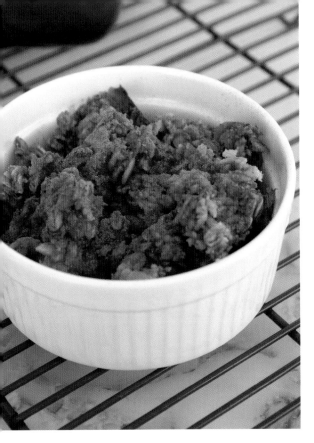

Baked Pumpkin Oatmeal

Cooked oats replenish your iron stores, while pumpkin provides vitamin A, fiber, and antioxidants.

Serves: 9 | Prep time: 10 minutes |
Cook time: 30 minutes

DRY INGREDIENTS

2 cups old-fashioned oats

½ teaspoon baking powder

¼ teaspoon salt

1 teaspoon ground cinnamon

1 teaspoon nutmeg

¼ teaspoon cloves

4 tablespoons ground flaxseeds

2 tablespoons chia seeds

WET INGREDIENTS

1½ cups milk of choice

1 cup pumpkin puree

¼ cup maple syrup

2 eggs

crushed walnuts, to top

1. Preheat the oven to 350°F.

2. In a medium bowl, combine the dry ingredients.

3. In a separate medium bowl, whisk together the milk, pumpkin, syrup, and eggs.

4. Combine the wet ingredients with the dry ingredients and stir to fully combine.

5. Pour the mixture into a greased 8 x 8-inch casserole pan.

6. Place the pan in the oven for 30 minutes, until the center of the baked oatmeal is set.

7. Cut into squares for serving.

8. Top with walnuts, if desired.

#MomHack: Making a batch of this baked oatmeal provides meals for several days in a row. Oatmeal will keep in the fridge for 5 days. Combine with milk to reheat and top with a dose of healthy fat to provide you with steady energy for hours. Oatmeal and flaxseeds included in the recipe are both well-known galactagogues, which are plant-derived substances that promote lactation.

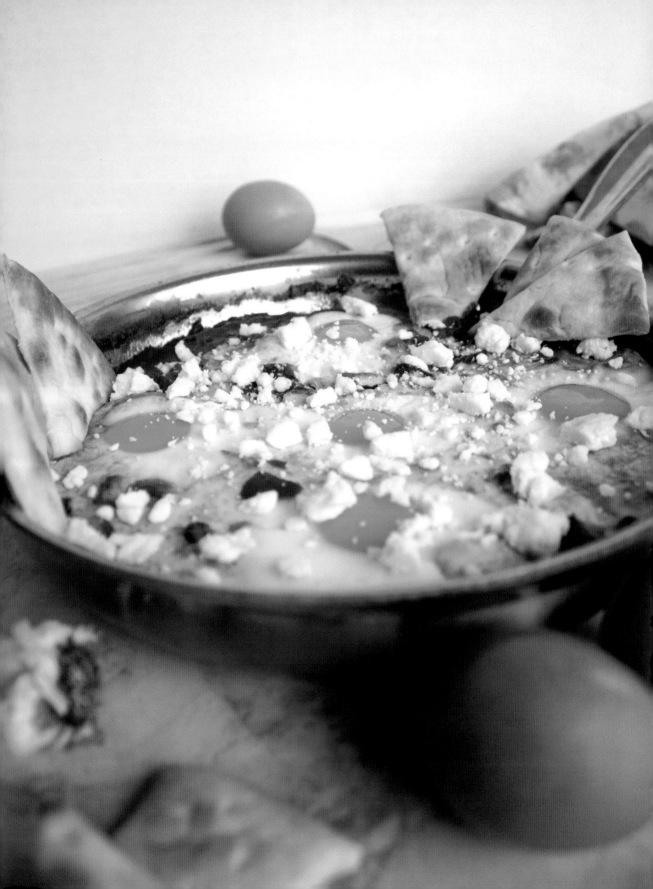

Shakshuka

Shakshuka, whose origin remains largely debated, is a common staple of Middle Eastern cuisine. Not only does it have a beautiful presentation, it embodies just what new moms need—warming spices to promote optimal digestion, protein to provide sustenance, and a whole lot of flavor.

Serves: 5 | Prep time: 10 to 15 minutes | Cook time: 15 minutes

INGREDIENTS

1 tablespoon extra-virgin olive oil

½ medium yellow onion, diced

3 cloves garlic, diced

1 (28-ounce) can diced tomatoes

1 teaspoon paprika

1 teaspoon ground cumin

½ teaspoon salt

¼ teaspoon chipotle chili powder

5 eggs

¼ cup crumbled feta cheese

fresh chopped parsley, to garnish

diced avocado, to garnish

pita or toasted baguette, to serve

1. Preheat the oven to 350°F.

2. In a large ovenproof or cast-iron sauté pan, heat the olive oil over medium heat.

3. Add the onion and garlic and sauté for 3 to 4 minutes until fragrant and browned.

4. Add the diced tomatoes, including juice, paprika, cumin, salt, and chipotle chili powder, and stir to combine.

5. Bring the tomato mixture to a simmer, stirring occasionally until the sauce thickens, about 10 minutes.

6. Once the sauce is thickened, create five wells in the sauce using the back of a wooden spoon and crack the eggs into each of these wells.

7. Place the pan in the oven and bake for 10 to 12 minutes until the egg is set and cooked throughout.

8. Let the pan cool and top with feta cheese, fresh parsley, and diced avocado, if desired. Serve with warm pita or baguette to dip in the sauce.

#MomHack: The ingredients included in this recipe are usually staple items kept on hand and the eggs are baked versus poached as they are prepared traditionally to help save time. Feel free to experiment with variations of spices and toppings as this is a great base recipe to build from.

Easy Egg Bites

Eggs, also known as nature's perfect food, are packed with protein, choline, and omega-3 fatty acids. This recipe pairs iron-rich spinach with tomato, rich in vitamin C, to boost iron absorption. But the toppings for these bites are really endless!

Serves: 6 | Prep time: 10 minutes | Cook time: 20 minutes

INGREDIENTS

6 eggs

¼ cup milk

½ cup shredded cheese of choice (mozzarella, cheddar, or pepper jack all work well)

1 cup fresh spinach

1 Roma tomato, chopped

¼ teaspoon salt

¼ teaspoon pepper

1. Preheat the oven to 350°F.

2. In a large mixing bowl, whisk together the eggs, milk, and cheese until blended.

3. In a small sauté pan, sauté the spinach and tomato together until the spinach is wilted, about 5 minutes. Add the sauté mixture to the eggs in the mixing bowl and stir to combine.

4. Spray a 12-cup muffin pan with cooking spray and pour the mixture into the cups, filling them two-thirds of the way full.

5. Place the muffin pan in the oven and bake for 20 minutes until fully cooked. There should be no runny egg yolks, and a toothpick inserted should come out clean.

#MomHack: Once you make a batch of these bites, you can easily assemble breakfast sandwiches by placing an egg bite between a grain of your choice (think English muffin, whole grain toast, or a tortilla) to have ready to warm up for early mornings.

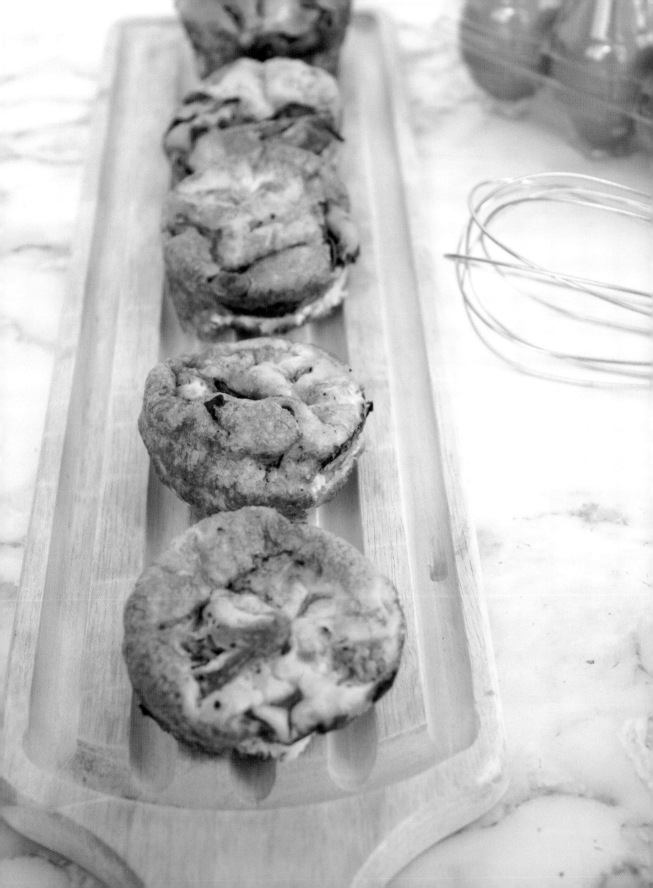

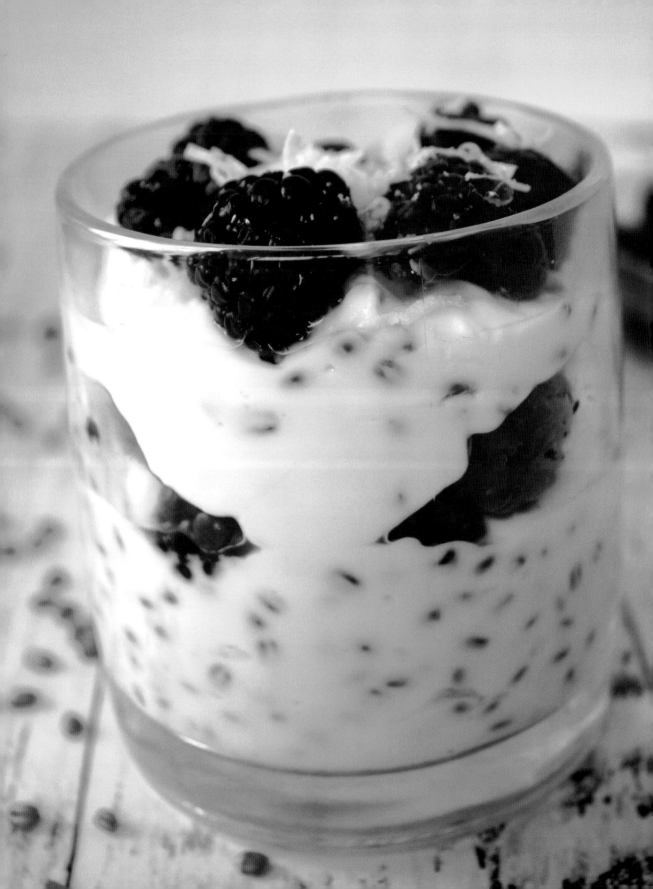

Wheat Berry Yogurt Parfaits

Wheat berries are a great way to add some variety to your mix of carbohydrates. Since wheat berries include all parts of the grain (bran, germ, and endosperm), they maintain a great amount of fiber, protein, and micronutrients and provide a wonderful, chewy texture.

Serves: 2 | Prep time: 5 minutes | Cook time: 20 minutes

INGREDIENTS

½ cup wheat berries

1½ cups water

dash of salt

6 ounces plain yogurt

1 cup mixed berries

½ cup granola

4 tablespoons chopped walnuts or nuts of choice

honey, coconut, dried fruit, or toppings of choice, to garnish

1. To cook the wheat berries, place them in a saucepan with the water and salt.

2. Bring the wheat berries to a boil, reduce to a simmer, covered with a lid, for about 20 minutes.

3. Check for doneness by spooning out a few wheat berries. They should be chewy and tender.

4. Once the wheat berries are done cooking, drain them from the saucepan.

5. Divide the yogurt in half and combine it with the cooked wheat berries, splitting the mixture between 2 serving glasses and layering the yogurt/wheat berry mixture in the bottoms of the bowls.

6. Add the mixed berries to both yogurt bowls to create a middle layer and top with the remaining plain yogurt.

7. Add the granola and walnuts to top and any other remaining toppings as desired.

#MomHack: Cooking the wheat berries is more of a time investment than popping Minute Rice in the microwave. However, the investment can be harvested in just how versatile the grain is. Make a batch of this grain and use it in soups, salads, desserts (puddings and yogurts), or swap it in for your normal grain rotation.

Sweet Potato Breakfast Bowl

Sweet potatoes, the vibrant root vegetable, now appear for not only lunch and dinner but also for breakfast! Since sweet potatoes contain carbohydrates, fiber, and antioxidants, they make a great item to swap into the breakfast rotation. Simply pair them with some protein and load them with your favorite sweet or savory toppings.

Serves: 2 | Prep time: 10 minutes | Cook time: 40 to 45 minutes

INGREDIENTS

2 medium sweet potatoes, halved lengthwise

1 cup plain full-fat Greek yogurt

2 tablespoons nut butter of choice

1 cup mixed berries

½ cup granola

honey, to top

1. Preheat the oven to 425°F. Lightly oil a baking sheet with cooking spray or olive oil.

2. Place the sweet potatoes flesh-side down on baking sheet and bake until tender, about 40 to 45 minutes. Remove the potatoes from the oven and allow them to cool on the baking sheet.

3. In each serving bowl place 1 baked potato, ½ cup of Greek yogurt, 1 tablespoon of nut butter, ½ cup of berries, and ¼ cup of granola, then top with honey as desired.

#MomHack: Roasting sweet potatoes in a batch lends to multiple possibilities for all meals of the day. Add them to breakfast bowls, mash them up to serve as a side, or even slice and top with nut butter or avocado for a nutrient-dense snack.

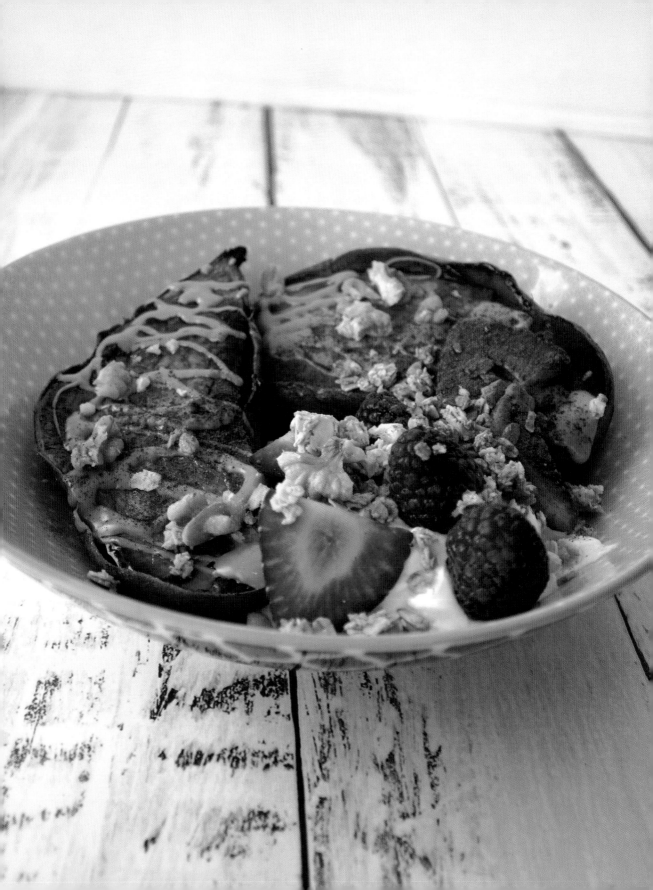

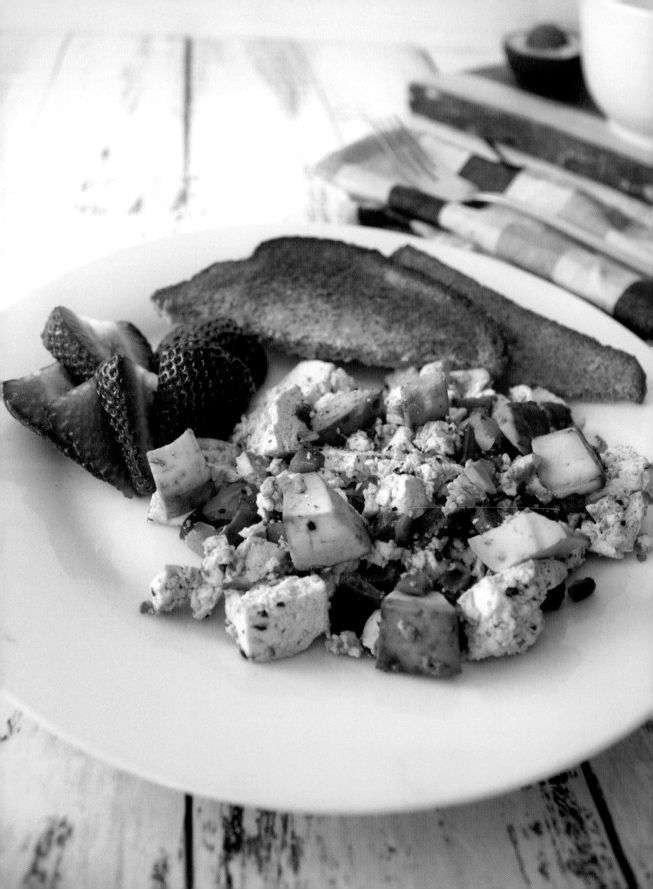

Tofu Scramble

Tofu gets dressed up in this quick breakfast dish. While tofu is typically used in stir-fries or other vegetarian dishes, in this recipe tofu serves as a great source of plant-based protein for breakfast. While the profile looks similar to eggs, adding in tofu to your breakfast rotation can provide a great source of protein and calcium. Since tofu is soybean based, the dish is rich in isoflavones, known for having a protective effect on cardiovascular health.

Serves: 4 | Prep time: 15 minutes | Cook time: 10 minutes

INGREDIENTS

1 block firm tofu

1 tablespoon olive oil

1 bell pepper (color of choice), seeded and diced

½ small red onion, diced

salt and pepper, to taste

1 teaspoon ground turmeric

¼ teaspoon garlic powder

1 medium avocado, diced

1. Place the tofu on a work surface. Place paper towels or a dish towel on top of the tofu block, then place a weight (such as a skillet) on top to allow the water to drain from the tofu. Leave the weight in place for about 10 minutes.

2. Once all liquid has drained from the tofu block, cut the tofu into 1-inch cubes.

3. Heat a medium skillet over medium heat with the olive oil.

4. Add the diced bell pepper, onion, salt, and pepper and sauté until the vegetables are softened, about 3 to 5 minutes.

5. Add in the tofu and, using a spatula, break it down into smaller pieces, and cook for about 5 minutes.

6. Add the turmeric, garlic powder, and additional salt and pepper, if desired, and stir to combine, allowing ingredients to simmer for 2 to 3 minutes.

7. Remove the tofu mixture from the pan and top with diced avocado.

#MomHack: Tofu can be a quick-and-easy protein to keep on hand for weeknight meals, since it cooks faster than animal protein. In this recipe, feel free to use up any vegetables you have on hand.

Chicken Sausage Breakfast Burritos

Burritos make a great postpartum meal, as they can load you up on nutrients and you can eat them with one hand! These burritos are packed with protein, zinc, potassium, and fiber from the chicken sauce, eggs, and beans, topped with sautéed vegetables and cheese for equal parts flavor and nutrition. To jazz up the flavor you can add in your favorite salsa or hot sauce and top with avocado upon serving.

Serves: 6 | Prep time: 15 minutes | Cook time: 15 to 20 minutes

INGREDIENTS

1 tablespoon olive oil

1 pound chicken sausage, casings removed

8 eggs

¼ cup milk

salt and pepper, to taste

2 bunches green onions, sliced

2 medium tomatoes, diced

6 large flour or wheat tortillas

2 (15-ounce) cans black beans, drained

2 cups shredded cheddar cheese

avocado, cilantro, sour cream, and salsa, to garnish

1. Heat the olive oil in a medium skillet over medium heat. Add the sausage, using a spatula to break apart the meat. Cook until all of the pieces are evenly browned, about 8 to 10 minutes.

2. While the sausage cooks, crack the eggs into a medium mixing bowl and whisk them together with the milk, adding salt and pepper to taste.

3. Once the sausage has cooked thoroughly, add the whisked eggs to the skillet, using a spatula to gently turn the eggs and scramble them until set, about 3 to 5 minutes.

4. Stir in the green onions and diced tomato to combine with the egg and sausage mixture, about 2 minutes, and then remove the skillet from heat.

5. Lay the tortillas on a work surface and place about ½ cup of black beans in the middle of each tortilla.

6. Top the beans with about ½ cup of the egg and sausage mixture. Add ¼ cup of cheese to each tortilla.

7. To wrap a burrito, fold in opposite sides of the tortilla tightly and place the burrito seam-side down on the work surface.

8. If serving immediately, cut the burrito in half and top with avocado, cilantro, sour cream, and salsa, as desired.

#MomHack: These burritos freeze and batch-cook well. To freeze burritos to serve later, cover each burrito tightly in plastic wrap or aluminum foil to seal, and place in a sealed freezer bag. When ready to eat, unwrap a burrito and warm it in the microwave for about 5 minutes, until heated throughout.

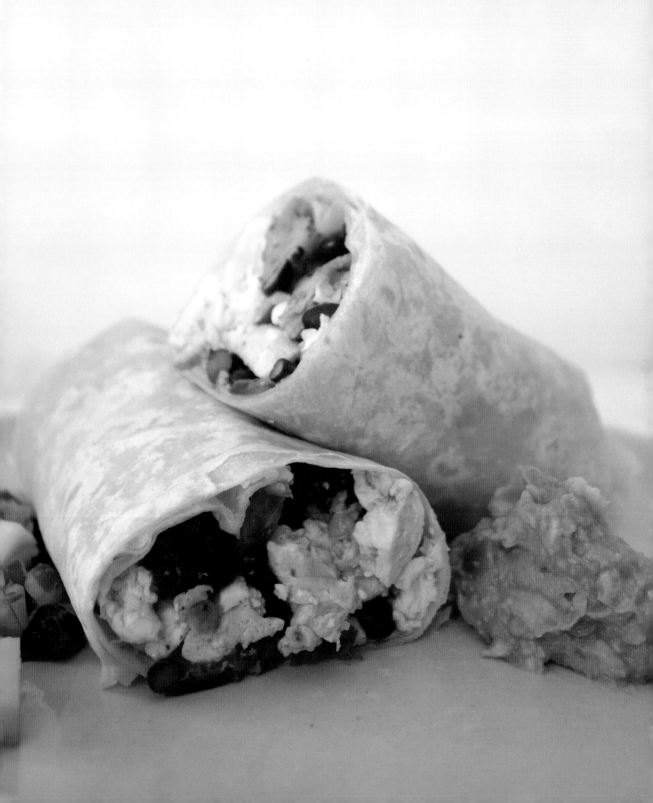

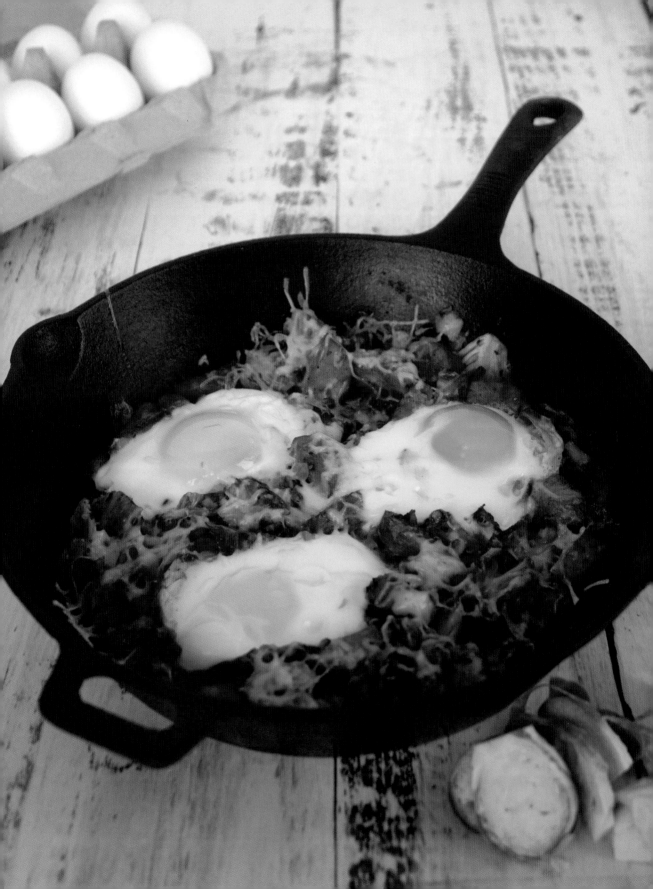

Brussels Sprout Breakfast Hash

Brussels sprouts make a debut at breakfast in this simple hash. Brussels sprouts are a cruciferous vegetable and are essentially miniature cabbages rich in fiber, vitamin K, and choline. Combined with chicken apple sausage and a sprinkle of gouda cheese, this recipe packs in great flavor as well.

Serves: 3 to 4 | Prep time: 15 minutes | Cook time: 20 minutes

INGREDIENTS

1½ tablespoons olive oil, divided

2 cloves garlic, minced

2 cups brussels sprouts, ends sliced and cut into thin slices

8 ounces chicken apple sausage links, sliced lengthwise and then into semicircles

3 eggs

4 ounces gouda cheese, shredded

1. In a medium skillet, heat 1 tablespoon of olive oil over medium heat.

2. Add the garlic to the skillet and heat until fragrant, around 3 to 4 minutes.

3. Add the brussels sprouts to the skillet and sauté until tender, about 5 minutes. Add the remaining ½ tablespoon of olive oil to help the sprouts tenderize.

4. Add the sausages to the skillet to cook with the brussels sprouts for another 5 minutes until both the brussels sprouts and the sausage are lightly browned.

5. Create 3 small holes in the skillet and crack the eggs into these holes to cook. Cover the skillet with a lid for about 4 to 5 minutes to cook the eggs.

6. Turn the heat off and add shredded cheese to top until melted. Serve warm.

#MomHack: Breakfast hashes are a great way to use vegetables or potatoes from dinner leftovers the night before. Simply sauté in the pan, add vegetables of choice, and throw an egg on top to make a nutritious and satisfying breakfast (or brunch!).

Turkey Patties with Apple and Fennel

Fennel has been a long-standing medicinal herb. In breastfeeding women, it has been associated with boosting milk production. Regardless of whether you are breastfeeding or not, integrating this herb postpartum provides a boost of antioxidants and adds a wonderful flavor to these turkey patties. The skin of the apple in this recipe is maintained during shredding to add fiber to the mix alongside turkey, which provides a great source of protein and B vitamins.

Serves: 8 | Prep time: 5 minutes | Cook time: 10 minutes

INGREDIENTS

1 pound ground turkey

1 tablespoon ground fennel seeds

1 teaspoon garlic powder

½ teaspoon salt

½ teaspoon pepper, to taste

1 Honeycrisp or Fuji apple with skin on, shredded

cooking spray or olive oil

1. In a medium bowl, combine the ground turkey with the fennel seeds, garlic powder, salt, and pepper

2. Add the apple to the ground turkey mixture.

3. Using a spatula, combine the ingredients together gently, being sure not to overmix.

4. Using a spoon, scoop about 2 tablespoons of turkey mixture from the bowl and roll in your hands to form a ball. Pat the mixture down to reduce thickness, forming a small patty, and set it aside on a plate. Repeat with the remaining turkey mixture.

5. Heat a medium cast-iron skillet over medium heat and coat with cooking spray or olive oil.

6. Place 4 to 5 patties at a time in the skillet to cook in batches, cooking them for 3 to 4 minutes on each side. Repeat until all patties have been cooked.

7. Patties are fully cooked when their internal temperature is 165°F. Serve warm immediately. To refrigerate patties for use in a later recipe, store in an airtight container for up to 3 days.

#MomHack: Making a batch of these provides versatile options to add to both meals and snacks throughout the week. These patties make a natural addition to breakfast; but they can also be served as a snack or even repurposed for dinner as sliders.

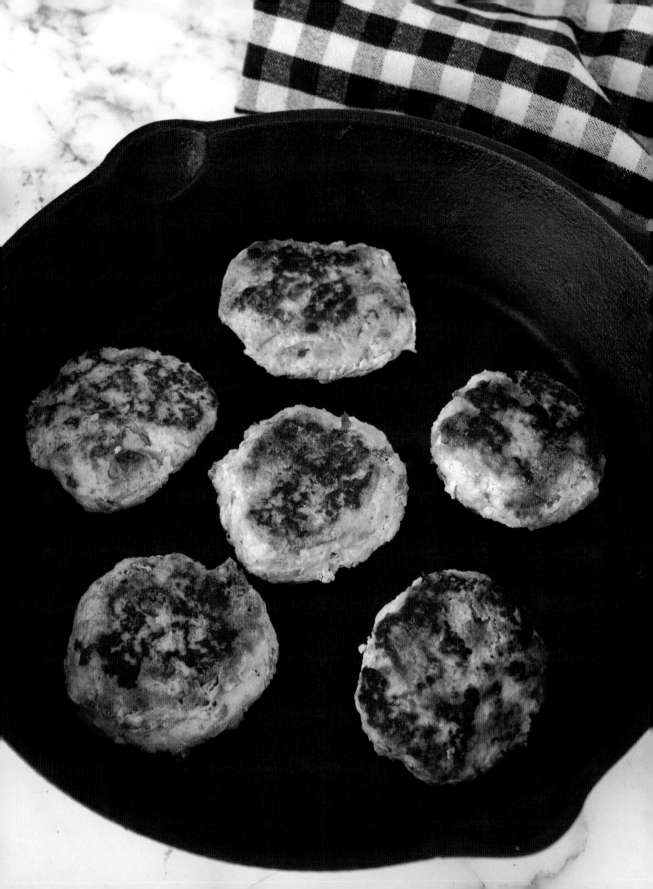

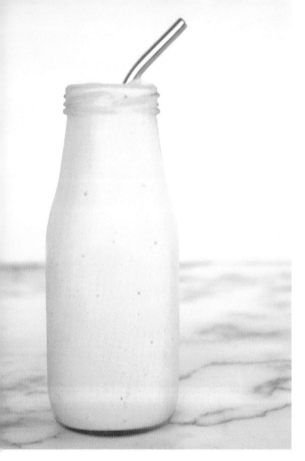

Glowing Green Smoothie

Avocado in a smoothie? Yes, the ever-versatile avocado not only makes for an amazing sandwich topping but also adds flavor, smooth texture, and nutrients to your morning smoothie. Ensuring that meals are rich in dietary fats is essential during postpartum recovery, as fats trigger the release of hormones that signal satiety and promote satisfaction to help you feel fuller longer.

Serves: 2 | Prep time: 5 minutes | Cook time: None

INGREDIENTS

1 ripe avocado, pitted, with skin removed

1 frozen banana, peeled and halved

1 cup milk of choice

1 tablespoon nut butter of choice

1 scoop vanilla or plain protein powder

1 cup ice

1. In a blender, combine all of the ingredients and puree until the mixture is smooth, about 1 to 2 minutes.

2. Pour the smoothie into 2 glasses and serve immediately.

#MomHack: Preventing avocados from becoming overripe tends to be tricky. If you have some that you notice are a day away from being overripe, you can pit them and freeze them to use in the smoothie. The frozen fruit and avocado make for a creamier texture in the smoothie.

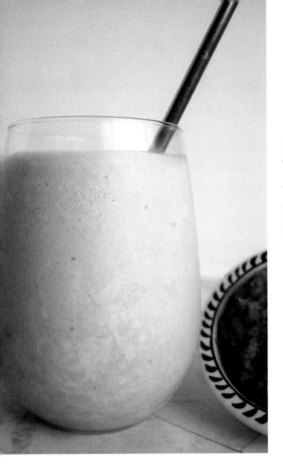

Pumpkin Smoothie

Pumpkin is the real all-star in this super-simple smoothie recipe. The pumpkin gets its rich orange color from beta-carotene, a carotenoid that the body converts into vitamin A, which provides a huge immunity boost for new moms. Pumpkin also provides a great source of fiber, vitamin C, vitamin E, and iron to boot.

Serves: 1 to 2 | Prep time: 3 minutes | Cook time: None

INGREDIENTS

½ cup pumpkin puree (not pumpkin pie filling)

1 frozen banana

1 scoop vanilla protein powder

¾ cup milk of choice

2 tablespoons ground flaxseeds

1 cup ice

1. Combine all of the ingredients in a blender.

2. Blend on high until the mixture combines and is smooth.

#MomHack: Keeping canned pumpkin puree on hand is great to add color, flavor, and nutrition to dishes. Add it to soups, stews, oatmeal, and smoothies for a creamy texture, or include it in baked goods.

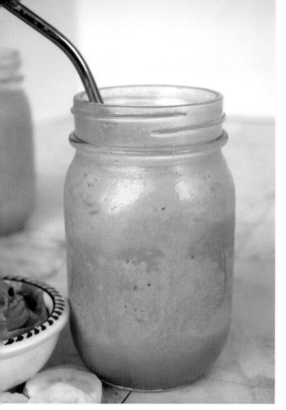

Peanut Butter Cup Smoothie

All the peanut butter cup taste with a helping of protein, fiber, and fat. The frozen banana makes the texture creamy and provides a great source of potassium as well!

Serves: 1 to 2 | Prep time: 5 minutes | Cook time: None

INGREDIENTS

1 frozen banana

1 8-ounce cup milk of choice

1 scoop chocolate protein powder

1 tablespoon ground flaxseeds

1 tablespoon peanut butter

½ cup ice

1. Combine all of the ingredients in a blender.

2. Blend on high until the mixture combines and is smooth.

#MomHack: Since liquids tend to empty faster from the stomach, adding a side of toast or blending in rolled oats to the smoothie can help delay emptying and provide satiety for longer.

Chapter 7

Lunch & Dinner

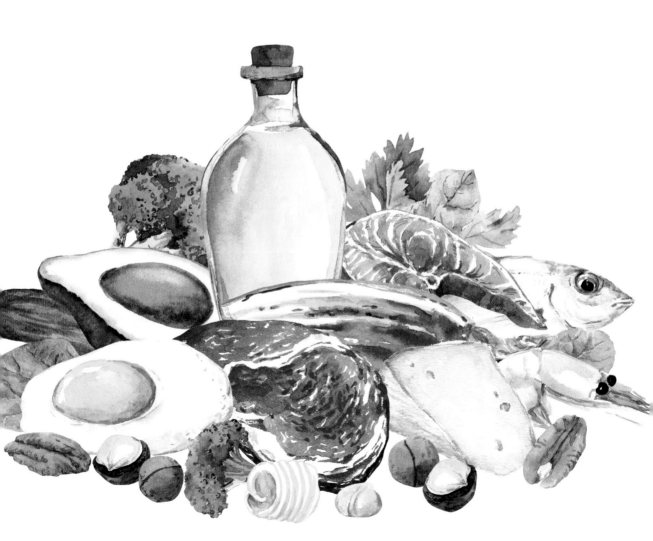

Split Pea Soup

Split pea soup provides all the comfort new moms need and packs in a powerful dose of B vitamins, folate, and thiamin, as well as a generous serving of fiber. When cooked, the beans break down to help provide a rich and creamy texture.

Serves: 6 to 8 | Prep time: 10 minutes | Cook time: 35 to 45 minutes

INGREDIENTS

2 tablespoon extra-virgin olive oil

1 medium yellow onion, diced

4 stalks celery, diced

2 large carrots, peeled and diced

2 cloves garlic, peeled and diced

2 cups split peas, rinsed

1 teaspoon salt, plus more to taste

1 teaspoon pepper, plus more to taste

8 cups broth (chicken or vegetable)

fresh shredded Parmesan, to serve

freshly cracked pepper, to serve

1. In a large Dutch oven or pot, heat the olive oil over medium heat.

2. Add the onion, celery, carrots, and garlic to the Dutch oven and sauté until the vegetables become tender and fragrant, about 3 to 4 minutes.

3. Add the split peas, salt, and pepper and stir to combine.

4. Add the broth and turn the heat up to medium-high to bring the mixture to a boil. Once the broth is at a boil, turn the heat down to low, cover the oven, and simmer the peas until they are tender, about 30 to 40 minutes. Add more broth or water to bring the soup to the desired texture or consistency.

5. Ladle the soup into bowls and top with shredded Parmesan cheese and pepper, if desired.

#MomHack: Legumes such as beans, peas, and nuts are essential postpartum staples for all new moms. Not only are they rich in protein, fat, and fiber, they are also cost-effective and can be stored in the pantry to have on hand for quick meals if making a grocery run is challenging (as life with a newborn very much is).

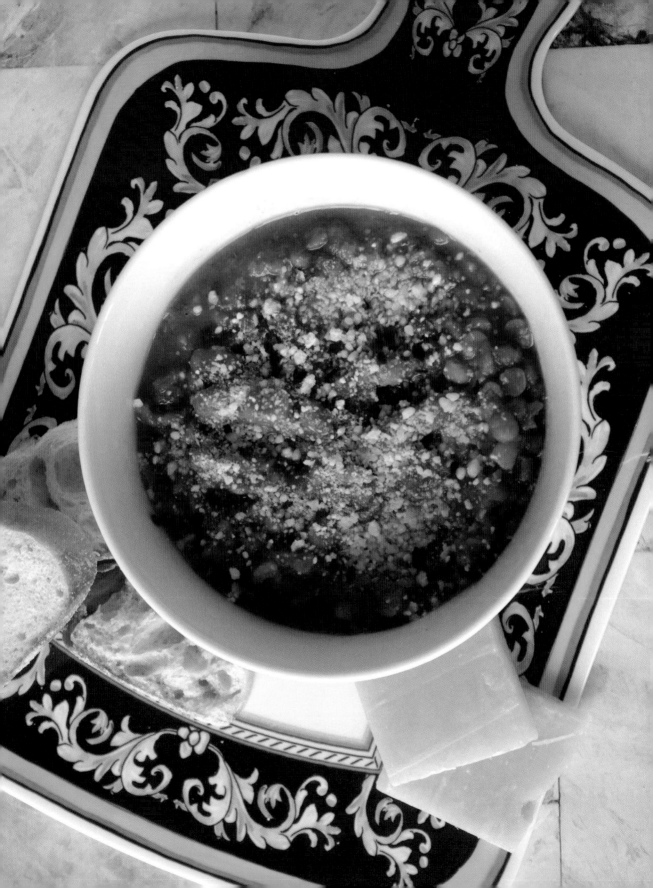

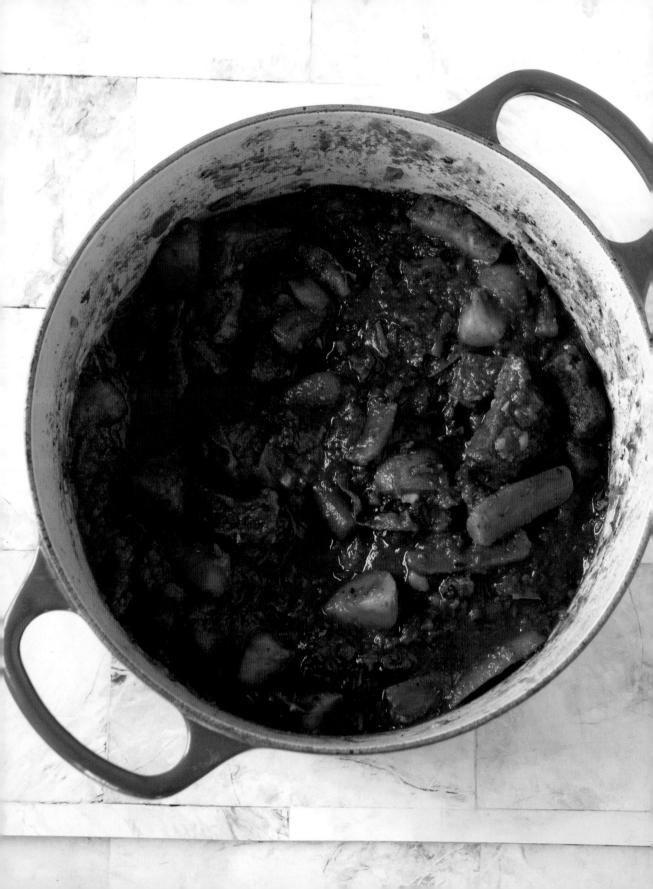

Beef Stew

Stew embodies all the goodness of a postpartum meal. It provides iron-rich beef, warm spices, and tender, well-cooked vegetables. Beef and animal proteins have been shown to have powerful recovery properties, as the iron in animal products is more readily available to replete stores that are diminished during birth.

Serves: 4 | Prep time: 20 minutes | Cook time: 1 to 1¼ hours

INGREDIENTS

1 tablespoon extra-virgin olive oil

1 medium yellow onion, diced

3 stalks celery, diced

2 to 3 large carrots, peeled and diced

3 to 4 cloves garlic, diced

1 teaspoon salt

1 teaspoon pepper

1 bay leaf

1 tablespoon Italian seasoning

1 pound beef stew meat

1 (14-ounce) can diced tomatoes

4 cups beef broth

2 cups baby red or Yukon potatoes, sliced in half

fresh parsley, to serve

1. In a large Dutch oven or pot, heat the olive oil over medium heat.

2. Add the onion, celery, carrots, and garlic and sauté until the vegetables are tender, about 3 to 4 minutes.

3. Add the salt, pepper, bay leaf, and Italian seasoning to the vegetables and stir to combine.

4. Remove the vegetable mixture to a separate large bowl.

5. Add the stew meat to the pot, ensuring that the pieces are not overcrowded. Brown the meat, about 5 minutes on each side.

6. Add the vegetables back to the pot with the meat. Add in the diced tomatoes and beef broth and bring the mixture to a boil.

7. Add the baby potatoes to the boiling stew mixture.

8. Once the liquid is boiling, cover the pot and bring the stew to a simmer to tenderize the meat. Cook for about 45 minutes to 1 hour.

9. Remove the bay leaf from the stew and serve with fresh parsley, as desired.

#MomHack: This recipe can be adapted for the slow cooker if you prefer to set it and forget it. You will need to complete the steps 1 to 5 to brown the vegetables and the meat. Then, add the rest of the ingredients (potatoes and liquid) to the slow cooker on low for 6 hours.

Slow Cooker Three Bean Chili

A good chili recipe is a mainstay for any household, and certainly in homes with a newborn. This recipe is simple enough to build upon and provides plenty of room for creativity. Use any beans you have on hand, add in extra vegetables such as bell peppers, carrots, zucchini, or squash, and adapt the spices to your liking.

Serves: 6 to 8 | Prep time: 10 minutes | Cook time: 6 hours

INGREDIENTS

1 tablespoon extra-virgin olive oil

1 medium onion, diced

3 cloves garlic, diced

2 tablespoons chili powder

1 teaspoon ground cumin

½ teaspoon paprika

½ teaspoon salt

1 (14-ounce) can fire-roasted diced tomatoes (regular if you prefer less spice)

3 (14-ounce) cans beans of any variety (garbanzos, chili beans, black beans, pinto beans, kidney beans, or cannellini beans), rinsed and drained

1 cup corn kernels (fresh or frozen)

2 cups vegetable broth

cilantro, shredded cheese, sour cream, lime juice, and red onion, to garnish

1. Heat the olive oil in a small pan and add the diced onion and garlic, sautéing for 2 to 3 minutes until fragrant. Transfer cooked ingredients to a 6-quart slow cooker.

2. Add the remaining ingredients to the slow cooker, stirring the ingredients to combine, and cook on low for 6 hours.

3. Taste when done, adding more salt to taste. Ladle the chili into bowls and add toppings as desired.

#MomHack: Make a batch of this chili and eat it for days without getting bored. Add it to a baked potato or over a well-cooked grain such as rice or quinoa, or simply vary your toppings to create a different meal every time.

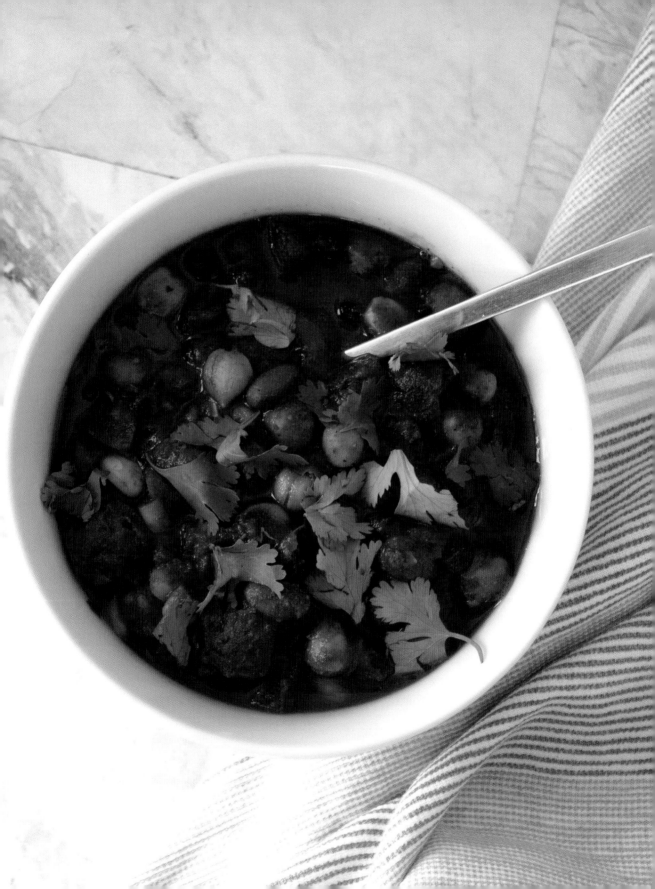

Lebanese Lentils

This dish is inspired by a traditional Lebanese dish, mujadara, which consists of lentils, rice, and crispy onions, alongside garlic and parsley. Simple ingredients provide flavor and deliver rich protein, iron, plant flavonoids, steady nutrients, and major staying power to new moms. This dish is best served warm and accompanied by some type of dip, such as hummus or tzatziki, to add another layer of flavor.

Serves: 4 to 6 | Prep time: 10 minutes | Cook time: 50 minutes

INGREDIENTS

2 tablespoons extra-virgin olive oil

1 medium yellow onion, thinly sliced

4 cloves garlic, minced

1 cup green or black lentils

1 cup cooked long-grain white rice

½ teaspoon salt

4 cups water

1 bunch fresh parsley, chopped

1. Heat the olive oil in a large sauté pot or Dutch oven over medium heat. Add the sliced onion and sauté until it is fragrant and golden-brown. Remove half for the topping and set it aside.

2. Add the minced garlic, lentils, and rice to the remaining onion in the pot, and stir to combine.

3. Add the salt and water to the pot and simmer, covered, for about 40 minutes, until the lentils and rice are tender and most of the liquid has been absorbed.

4. Top with fresh parsley and serve warm.

#MomHack: Keeping a supply of rice and dried or canned beans on hand provides a solid base for creating nourishing postpartum meals. These staples will serve to provide steady nutrition in the stretch between grocery runs.

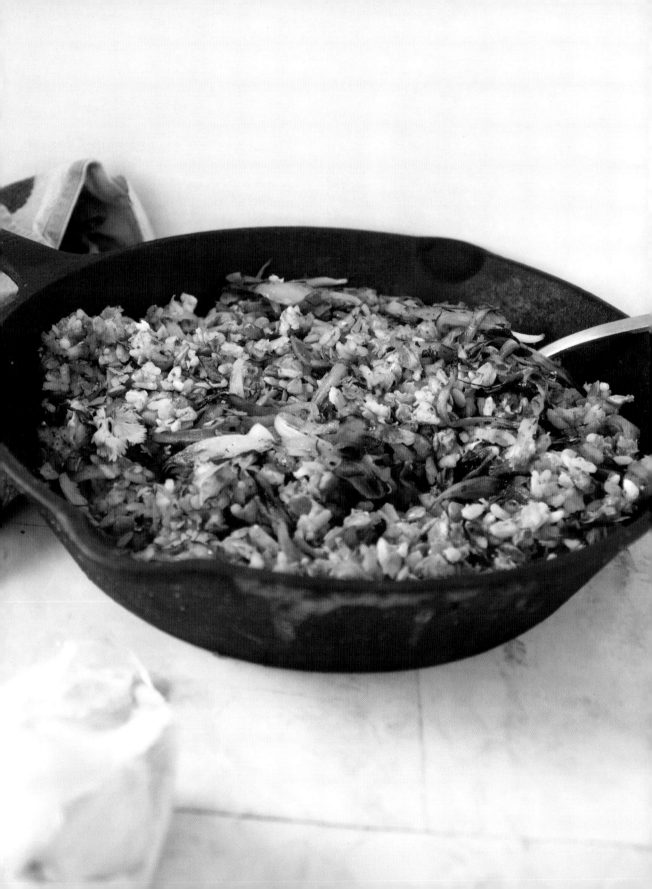

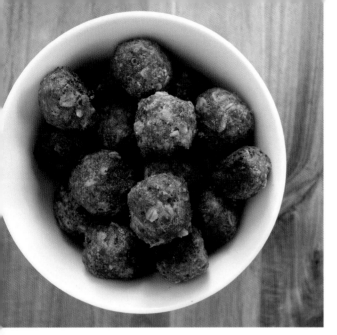

Baked Meatballs

Meatballs are a classic and flavorful item that adds sustenance and satisfaction. Almost every meatball recipe involves breadcrumbs to serve as a binder for the meat so the meatball does not fall apart. Ground oats take the place of breadcrumbs in this recipe, creating the same effect while adding a dash more fiber and iron to the mix. 80/20 ground beef tends to work best and provide the best flavor.

Serves: 6 | Prep time: 10 minutes | Cook time: 15 minutes

INGREDIENTS

1 pound ground beef

1 egg

¼ cup finely diced onion

½ cup finely ground rolled oats (you can leave some unground for more texture, if you like)

½ cup grated Parmesan cheese

2 teaspoons garlic powder

1 tablespoon Italian seasoning

1 teaspoon salt

1 teaspoon pepper

dash of red pepper flakes

½ cup 2% milk

1. Preheat the oven to 425°F and line a large baking sheet with parchment paper.

2. In a large mixing bowl, combine the ground beef, egg, onion, oats, cheese, and seasonings.

3. Slowly add the milk to the meat mixture. Use your hands to combine it and prevent overmixing, so that the seasoning is well distributed throughout.

4. Once all of the ingredients have been well mixed, use a large spoon to scoop the mixture, 1 tablespoon at a time, into your hands, rolling the meat between your palms to form a meatball.

5. Repeat step 4 with the remaining meat mixture.

6. Place the meatballs on the lined baking sheet and bake for 15 minutes, or until the meatballs reach an internal temperature of 165°F.

#MomHack: While meatballs are traditionally pan-fried, baking is a simpler and less time-intensive cooking method.

Caprese Pasta Salad

Simple, fresh ingredients combine to provide maximum flavor in this pasta salad recipe. When using few ingredients, it is best to try to source the freshest possible items. This not only boosts the flavor but also provides the most nutrition. Fresh herbs used in this recipe provide essential oils and plant polyphenols.

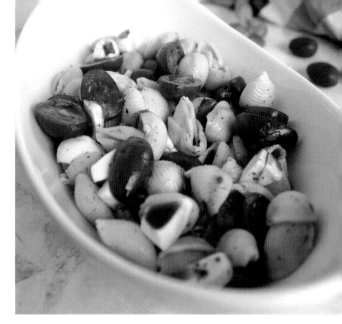

Serves: 4 | Prep time: 35 minutes |
Cook time: None

INGREDIENTS

8 ounces cherry mozzarella

8 ounces cherry tomatoes, halved

½ cup extra-virgin olive oil

4 cloves garlic, minced

2 tablespoons sun-dried tomatoes with oil, chopped

handful of fresh basil, minced

2 tablespoons fresh or dried parsley

½ teaspoon salt

½ teaspoon pepper

16 ounces cooked al dente pasta such as orecchiette or shells, chilled

balsamic glaze, to serve

chopped basil, to serve

1. In a medium mixing bowl, combine all of the ingredients except the pasta and stir to combine.

2. Place the tomato and mozzarella mixture in fridge, covered, for about 30 minutes or longer to allow the flavors to marinate.

3. Add the marinated tomato and mozzarella mixture to the al dente pasta and toss thoroughly to combine.

4. If desired, top the pasta with balsamic glaze and additional fresh basil.

5. Serve chilled or warm, if desired.

#MomHack: Pasta salad is a great way to use up leftover pasta and vegetables in the fridge. You can certainly mix and match ingredients to taste here; some options to rotate in include olives, red onion, bell peppers, pepperoncini, and feta. Balsamic glaze is available prepared in advance and is thicker than balsamic vinegar to add color and flavor to many dishes.

Black Bean and Sweet Potato Bake

I know that casseroles can feel a touch out of date, but this one is a perfect postpartum meal packed with goodness. Warming spices, ancient quinoa, and the perfect combination of sweet potatoes and black beans all come together with roasted vegetables and, of course, cheese.

Serves: 6 | Prep time: 25 minutes | Cook time: 45 minutes

INGREDIENTS

2 medium sweet potatoes, peeled and diced into small cubes

2 bell peppers, any color, diced

1 poblano pepper, diced

1 zucchini or squash, diced

1 medium yellow onion, diced

2 tablespoons canola or olive oil

½ teaspoon salt

½ teaspoon pepper

1½ teaspoons ground cumin

1 teaspoon garlic powder

1 teaspoon paprika

1 tablespoon chili powder

¼ teaspoon cayenne pepper (optional)

2 cups corn kernels

1 (15-ounce) can black beans, rinsed and drained

1 cup cooked quinoa

1 (15-ounce) can red enchilada sauce

1½ cups shredded Mexican cheese

1. Preheat the oven to 425°F.

2. Add the sweet potatoes, peppers, squash, and onion to a large bowl and toss with the oil, salt and pepper, cumin, garlic powder, paprika, chili powder, and cayenne pepper, if desired, ensuring that all the vegetables are coated.

3. Place the mixture on a baking sheet and roast for 25 minutes, until the sweet potatoes are tender.

4. Remove the baking pan from the oven and place all of the cooked vegetables in a medium bowl. Add the corn, black beans, and cooked quinoa to the mixture and combine.

5. Add the enchilada sauce to the mixture and toss to coat completely with the sauce.

6. Transfer the ingredients to a 9 x 13-inch casserole dish and top with cheese.

7. Cover with foil and bake in the oven for 20 minutes, or until the cheese is melted and bubbly.

#MomHack: This dish is hearty enough to serve on its own; however, ground beef, turkey, or shredded chicken can add additional protein. If you prefer milder flavors, you can omit the poblano pepper, but I find the flavor it adds to this dish is amazing. To save time, you can use frozen corn and peppers if needed; simply cook them according to package instructions and drain.

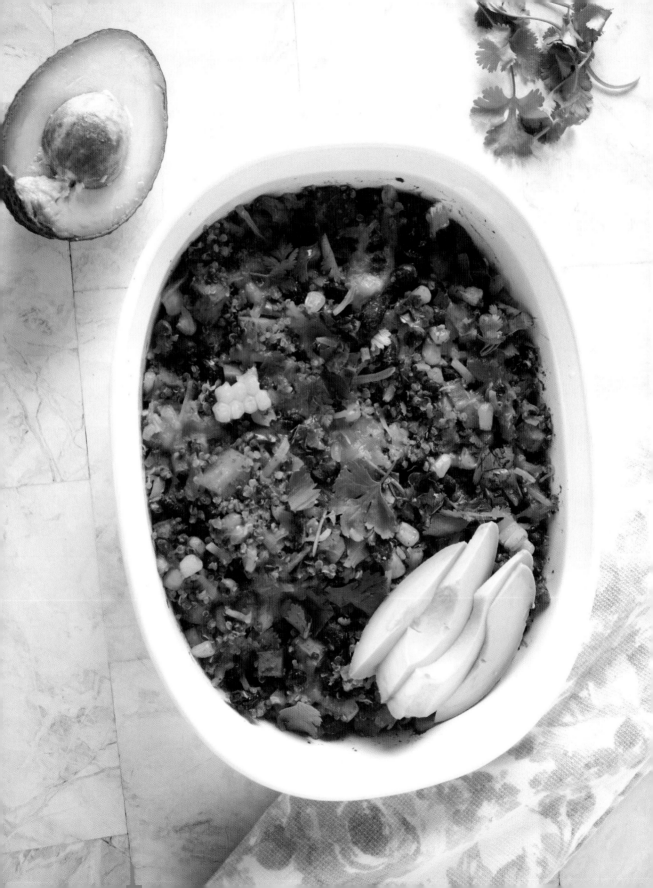

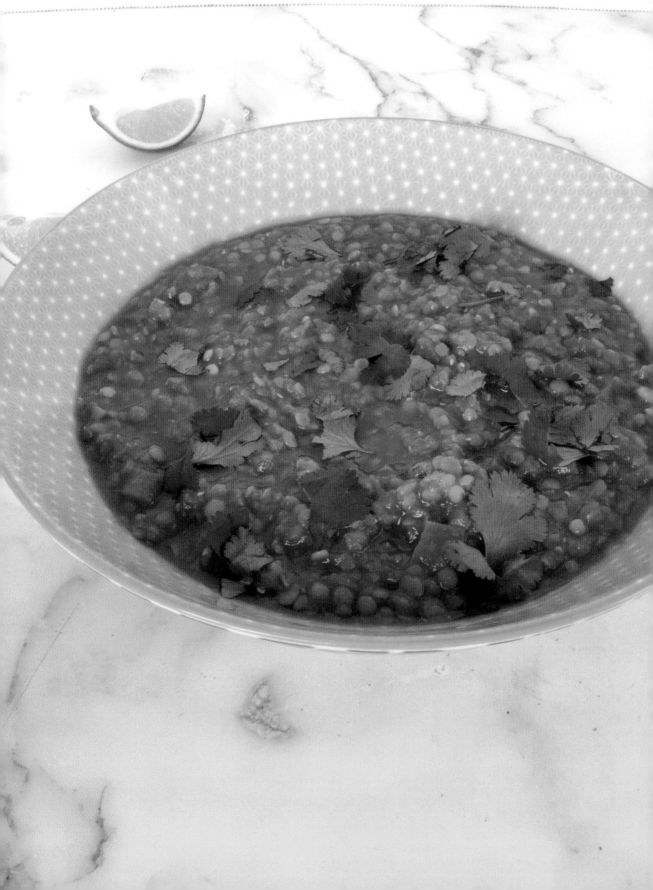

Golden Lentil Soup

Red lentils, tomato, ginger, and turmeric promote optimal digestion and healing. Ginger contains digestive enzymes and promotes optimal lactation. Combining the red lentils with tomato assists in the absorption of plant-derived iron to boost maternal iron status and provides essential protein to promote tissue healing.

Serves: 4 | Prep time: 15 minutes | Cook time: 6 hours

INGREDIENTS

½ medium yellow onion, diced

2 large carrots, peeled and diced

4 cloves garlic, minced

1½ cups dried red lentils

4 cups chicken broth

1 cup water

1 (6-ounce) can tomato paste

1 teaspoon salt

1 teaspoon pepper

3 teaspoons ground turmeric

1 teaspoon ground cumin

3 teaspoons fresh grated ginger

juice of 1 lime, to serve (optional)

chopped cilantro, to serve (optional)

plain yogurt, to serve (optional)

1. Place all of the ingredients into a 6-quart slow cooker and set on low for 6 hours, stirring to combine when finished.

2. To serve, ladle into bowls and top with fresh-squeezed lime, cilantro, and plain yogurt, if desired.

#MomHack: Simply dump the ingredients in the slow cooker to simmer aromatic spices throughout the day, and dish up a dose of soul-nourishing lentils. Warming foods assist mothers in restoring and healing the body after birth. You can keep ginger in the freezer to have on hand to use in recipes as needed. Store the root in a freezer-safe container. No need to thaw—just use what you need and return the rest to the freezer.

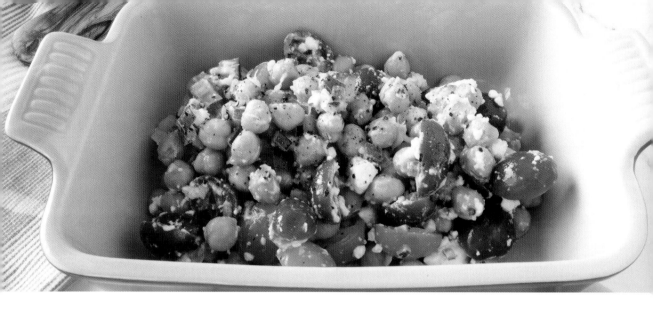

Garbanzo Bean Salad

Garbanzo beans are a rich source of folate, manganese, and fiber. They are also rich in bioactive plant compounds such as sterols, tannins, and polyphenols, all of which support heart health and reduce cholesterol. This bean salad upholds traditional Mediterranean flavors and is versatile for serving alongside a well-cooked grain, crackers, or on top of a bed of greens.

Serves: 4 | Prep time: 10 minutes | Cook time: None

INGREDIENTS

1 (15-ounce) can garbanzo beans, drained

½ cucumber, peeled and diced

¼ cup diced red onion

1 pint cherry tomatoes, halved

2 to 3 cloves garlic, minced

¼ cup crumbled feta cheese

1 tablespoon extra-virgin olive oil

salt and pepper, to taste

1. Pour the beans into a medium mixing bowl.

2. Add all of the chopped ingredients to the mixing bowl.

3. Incorporate the feta cheese and drizzle olive oil over the ingredients.

4. Add salt and pepper to taste.

#MomHack: Beans serve as a quick and nutrient-dense option for postpartum. While purchasing dried beans and soaking them can certainly be more cost-effective and provide optimal nutrition, canned beans are an ideal staple to have on hand. They provide a boost of protein to meals and can be added to salads or stews, or simply sautéed.

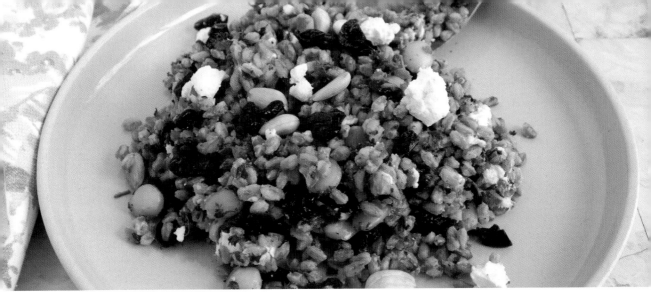

Moroccan Farro Salad

Farro is a wonderful ancient grain. I've added it to the rotation of whole grains in this cookbook for its lovely nutty flavor and chewy texture. While quinoa tends to steal the show as a protein-rich grain, farro packs a similar combination of protein and fiber, making it a superstar postpartum staple.

Serves: 2 | Prep time: 5 minutes | Cook time: 10 minutes

INGREDIENTS

2 cups cooked farro

¼ cup Marcona almonds

¼ cup dried cranberries

1 (2-ounce) package goat cheese, crumbled

2 tablespoons olive oil

1 bunch parsley, minced

½ teaspoon salt

½ teaspoon pepper

1. Cook the farro according to package instructions.

2. Place the farro in a medium bowl and add in the almonds, cranberries, cheese, olive oil, and parsley.

3. Combine the ingredients and season with salt and pepper.

4. Store in an airtight container to chill for 10 to 15 minutes, allowing the flavors to combine. Serve.

#MomHack: This grain-based salad is perfect for batch cooking. Divide it up into mason jars to have individual portions on hand. Simply add a protein source such as beans or chicken and you have a satisfying, nutrient-packed lunch. This salad also serves as a great base for experimenting. Try adding chopped dates or cherries in place of the cranberries or swapping out the almonds for a nut of your choice.

Roasted Tomato and Fennel Soup

Fennel is commonly known for supporting lactation postpartum. The herb boasts a licorice-like taste and is thought to mimic estrogen in the body. Combining this sweet-flavored herb with tomatoes (rich in vitamin C), sulfur-rich garlic, and onion provides a nutrient kick for moms.

Serves: 4 | Prep time: 15 minutes | Cook time: 40 minutes

INGREDIENTS

12 Roma tomatoes, ends cut and halved

1 head fennel, stalks and leaves removed, sliced

1 small yellow onion, sliced

4 cloves garlic

2 to 3 tablespoons olive oil

1 teaspoon salt

1 teaspoon pepper

1 cup vegetable stock

1 to 2 tablespoons heavy cream (optional)

1. Preheat the oven to 350°F.

2. Place the tomatoes on a large baking sheet lined with parchment paper.

3. Add the fennel and onion to the baking sheet with the tomatoes.

4. Add the whole garlic cloves to the baking sheet.

5. Drizzle the olive oil over the vegetables and toss with salt and pepper to thoroughly cover all the ingredients.

6. Place the baking sheet in the oven and roast the vegetables for 40 minutes, until caramelized.

7. Let vegetables cool briefly once removed from the oven, then add them to a blender with the stock. Blend together until smooth.

8. If you prefer a thicker and creamier soup, pour the mixture back into a pan on the stovetop, add 1 to 2 tablespoons of heavy cream, if desired, and stir.

#MomHack: Great made with vegetables that need to be used up, this soup serves as a great way to help clean out the fridge. Some other options that would work well include carrots, parsnips, and leeks. Simply chop them up and add them to the roasting pan. This soup's flavor is enough to stand independently. But you may add some cream or cheese for richness, if desired.

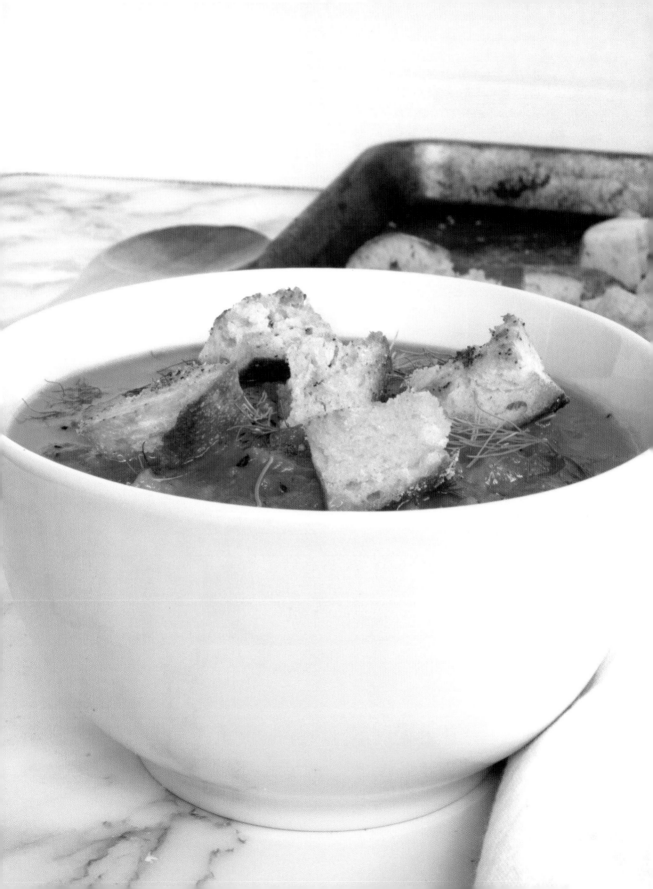

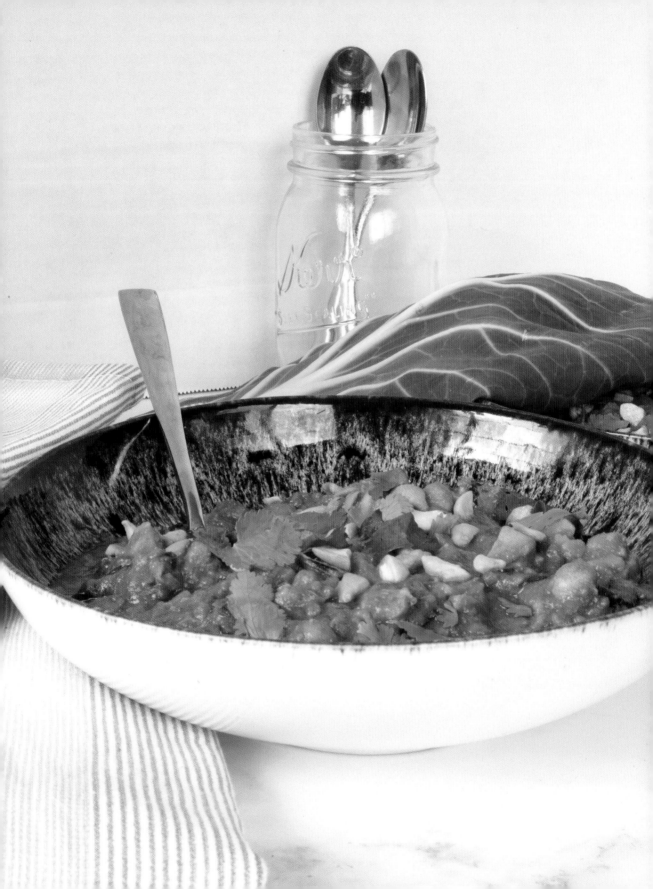

African Peanut Stew

This nourishing stew hosts several nutrient powerhouses. Ginger, garlic, onion, and jalapeño provide warming spice and rich flavor, and sweet potato and garbanzo beans add sustenance with complex carbohydrates and protein. If you are concerned about the spice level passing into your breastmilk, you can always adjust the amount of jalapeño. However, typically babies appreciate the unique and different flavors provided by the diversity of foods in the maternal diet.

Serves: 4 | Prep time: 15 minutes | Cook time: 20 minutes

INGREDIENTS

1 tablespoon olive oil

1 small yellow onion, diced

1 small jalapeño pepper, diced, core and seeds removed

3 cloves garlic, minced

knob of fresh ginger, shredded to make 2 tablespoons

1 teaspoon ground cumin

1 teaspoon salt

dash of cayenne pepper

1 (6-ounce) can tomato paste

1 (14-ounce) can garbanzo beans, rinsed and drained

4 cups vegetable stock

1 large sweet potato, peeled and diced into cubes

½ cup natural peanut butter

1 bunch collard greens, chopped

chopped cilantro, to serve

peanuts, to serve

[AU: Raw, cooked, whole?]

1. Heat the olive oil in a medium Dutch oven over medium heat.

2. Add the onion, jalapeño pepper, garlic, and ginger to the Dutch oven and sauté for 2 minutes, until fragrant

3. Add the cumin, salt, and cayenne pepper.

4. Add the tomato paste and garbanzo beans and stir to combine.

5. Pour in the vegetable stock and bring the heat up high.

6. Once the stock is boiling, add the sweet potato.

7. Let the mixture return to a boil, stir in the peanut butter, then reduce the heat and cover the pot and simmer for 15 minutes, or until the sweet potatoes are tender.

8. Stir in the collard greens until combined.

9. Top stew with chopped cilantro and peanuts, as desired, and serve.

#MomHack: This stew freezes well, so it would be a wonderful option to prepare in large batches to have on hand. Experiment with different combinations, such as swapping the beans for chicken, or kale for the collard greens.

Herb Baked Salmon

Touted for being a key source of omega-3 fatty acids, salmon makes a superstar postpartum meal. Omega-3 fatty acids, known for their myriad of health benefits, play a key role in supporting new moms by reducing symptoms of anxiety and depression as well as fighting off inflammation in the body.

Serves: 4 | Prep time: 10 minutes | Cook time: 12 to 15 minutes

INGREDIENTS

4 (6-ounce) salmon fillets (1-inch thickness)

3 to 4 cloves garlic, minced

1 bunch fresh parsley, minced

1 bunch fresh mint, minced

1 tablespoon extra-virgin olive oil

juice of 1 lemon

1 teaspoon salt

1 teaspoon pepper

1. Preheat the oven to 425°F.

2. Line a baking sheet with parchment paper and spray it with cooking spray.

3. Add the garlic, parsley, and mint to small bowl.

4. Add the olive oil and lemon juice to the bowl with the garlic mixture.

5. Stir the mixture and pour it over salmon fillets on the baking sheet.

6. Season each fillet with salt and pepper.

7. Bake for 12 to 15 minutes, until the internal temperature reaches 145°F (this will depend on the thickness of the salmon fillets).

#MomHack: Life with a newborn can be hectic. Thankfully, salmon fillets can be cooked from frozen, if desired. Using a sufficient amount of oil keeps the fillets moist when cooking; simply modify the recipe by using frozen fillets, adding the mixture of oil, garlic, and herbs, and baking!

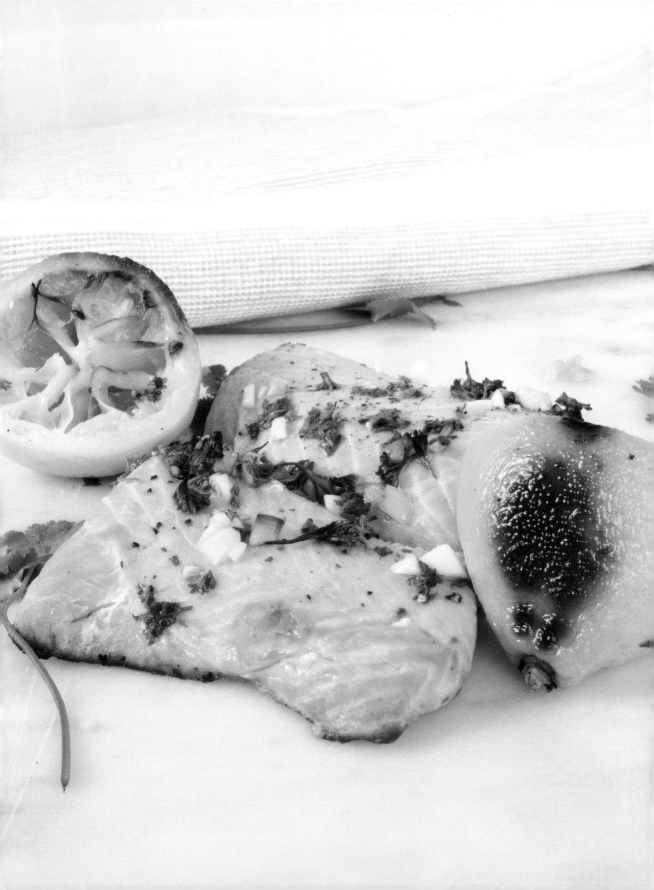

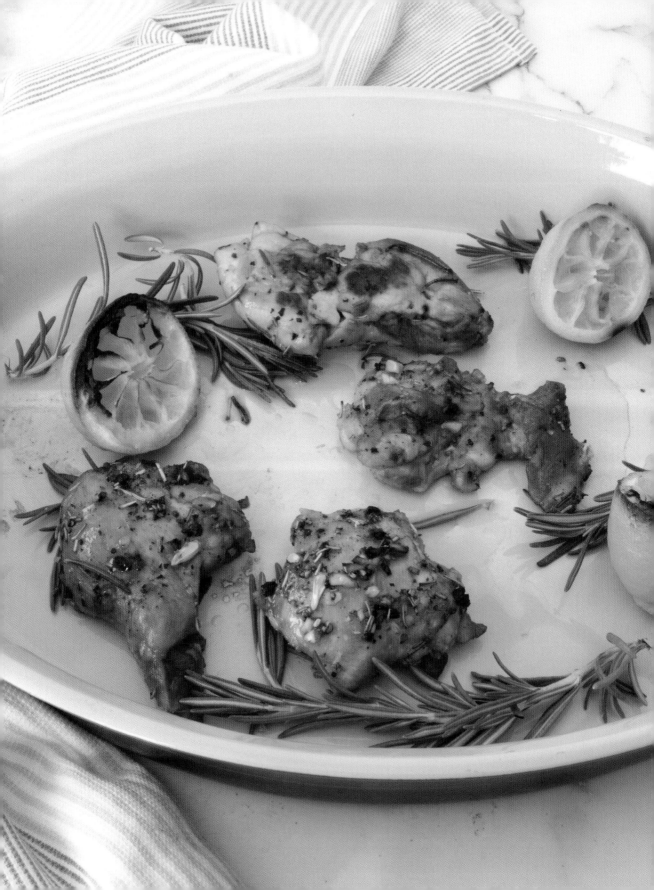

Lemon Baked Chicken

The versatility of chicken seems to be endless, and the high-quality protein it provides makes this dish essential for new moms. Rosemary paired with lemon provides delicious flavor and the herb itself has long been documented as a cognitive stimulant, a welcome benefit to sleep-deprived new moms. Chicken breasts can be substituted for the chicken thighs. However, chicken thighs tend to retain more of the classic Mediterranean flavors used in this recipe. To infuse even more rich flavor, consider marinating the dish the night before.

Serves: 4 | Prep time: 10 minutes | Cook time: 25 to 30 minutes

INGREDIENTS

2 tablespoons extra-virgin olive oil, plus more to serve

3 to 4 cloves garlic, minced

3 to 4 sprigs fresh rosemary

juice of 1 lemon

1 pound boneless chicken thighs

½ teaspoon salt, plus more to taste

½ teaspoon pepper

sliced lemons, to serve

fresh rosemary, to serve

1. Preheat the oven to 400°F. Combine the olive oil, minced garlic, rosemary, and lemon juice in a bowl and stir to combine.

2. Place the chicken thighs on a rimmed baking sheet and pour the olive oil mixture over each chicken thigh.

3. Season each chicken thigh with salt and pepper.

4. Place the baking sheet in the oven, uncovered, and bake for 25 to 30 minutes, depending on the thickness of the chicken thigh. The chicken is cooked thoroughly when the juices run clear and the internal temperature has reached 165°F. Allow chicken to rest on baking sheet for 5 minutes.

5. To serve, place chicken on a large platter with sliced lemons, fresh rosemary, and a drizzle of olive oil, if desired.

#MomHack: Batch-cook this meal and keep leftovers on hand to have a tasty protein-packed option you can use on top of salads and in wraps.

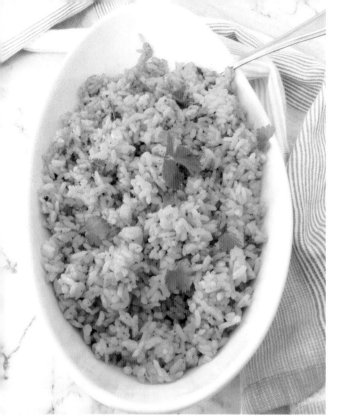

Yellow Rice

Turmeric turns regular white rice into a nutrition goldmine. Not only does the turmeric add a gorgeous color to the dish, but curcumin, the active ingredient in turmeric, can boost brain function.

Serves: 10 | Prep time: 10 minutes | Cook time: 20 minutes

INGREDIENTS

1 cup short-grain white rice

1 cup water

1 cup chicken stock

2 tablespoon extra-virgin olive oil

½ small onion, diced

1 teaspoon ground turmeric

1 teaspoon garlic powder

1 teaspoon pepper

1 teaspoon salt

1. Combine all of the ingredients in a rice cooker and cook on rice setting until done, about 20 minutes.

#MomHack: This dish pairs well with the Lemon Baked Chicken (page 75) or Herb Baked Salmon (page 72). Leftovers from a batch of this recipe can also be repurposed in endless possibilities, such as stir-fries, bowls, or wraps.

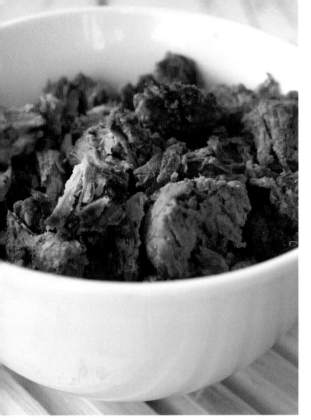

Easy Shredded Beef

Not only is beef rich in protein and iron, it is also rich in vitamins and minerals such as zinc, selenium, and B vitamins that assist with repletion postpartum.

Serves: 4 | Prep time: 10 minutes | Cook time: 8 hours

INGREDIENTS

1 pound beef stew meat (small to medium-size pieces)

½ cup beef broth

½ tablespoon kosher salt

½ tablespoon garlic powder

freshly cracked pepper, to taste

1. Place the stew meat and broth in a slow cooker.

2. Distribute the salt, garlic powder, and black pepper evenly over the meat.

3. Cover the slow cooker and cook on low for 8 hours until the beef shreds easily with a fork.

4. Mix the shredded meat with the broth, top with freshly cracked pepper, and serve.

#MomHack: One pot and multiple possibilities for this shredded beef. Make a batch to serve over your favorite cooked grain, in tacos, or with simple sides. You can buy the beef stew meat already diced into medium-size pieces to really save time.

White Bean and Chicken Soup

This soup marries the traditional flavors of a Tuscan white bean soup with chicken. The combination of carrot, celery, and onion (known as mirepoix) provides protein sustenance, a rich aroma, and a dose of antioxidants. The use of white beans adds creaminess and texture as well as fiber, folate, and magnesium.

Serves: 4 to 6 | Prep time: 10 minutes | Cook time: 30 to 35 minutes

INGREDIENTS

½ medium yellow onion, diced

2 medium carrots, peeled and diced

2 stalks celery, diced

2 cloves garlic, diced

1 teaspoon salt

¼ teaspoon pepper

1 teaspoon dried thyme

1 (15-ounce) can cannellini beans, drained

1 quart chicken broth

16 ounces whole chicken breast

Parmesan rind (optional)

French baguette, cubed, to serve

1. Heat a Dutch oven with olive oil over medium heat.

2. Add the carrots, celery, onion, and garlic to the Dutch oven and sauté for 3 to 4 minutes, until the vegetables are fragrant and tender.

3. Add the salt, pepper, thyme, cannellini beans, and broth to the Dutch oven and stir.

4. Allow the mixture to come to a boil, then add the chicken breast, allowing chicken to cook.

5. Boil the chicken for 10 to 12 minutes until fully cooked, then reduce the heat to a simmer and cover the Dutch oven, stirring occasionally.

6. Simmer the soup for 10 to 15 minutes, using a wooden spoon to press the white beans along the side of the Dutch oven to thicken the soup. The chicken should start to fall apart into large chunks; use two forks to shred larger pieces into smaller bites.

7. Add Parmesan rind to the soup, if desired. Serve in bowls, topped with cubed French baguette.

#MomHack: Smashing the white beans along the side of the pan is essential for increasing the thickness of the soup and creating a great texture. This soup freezes well for up to 3 months, just be sure to let it cool completely before sealing and storing it in the freezer to prevent large ice crystals forming and ruining the texture of the soup when reheating.

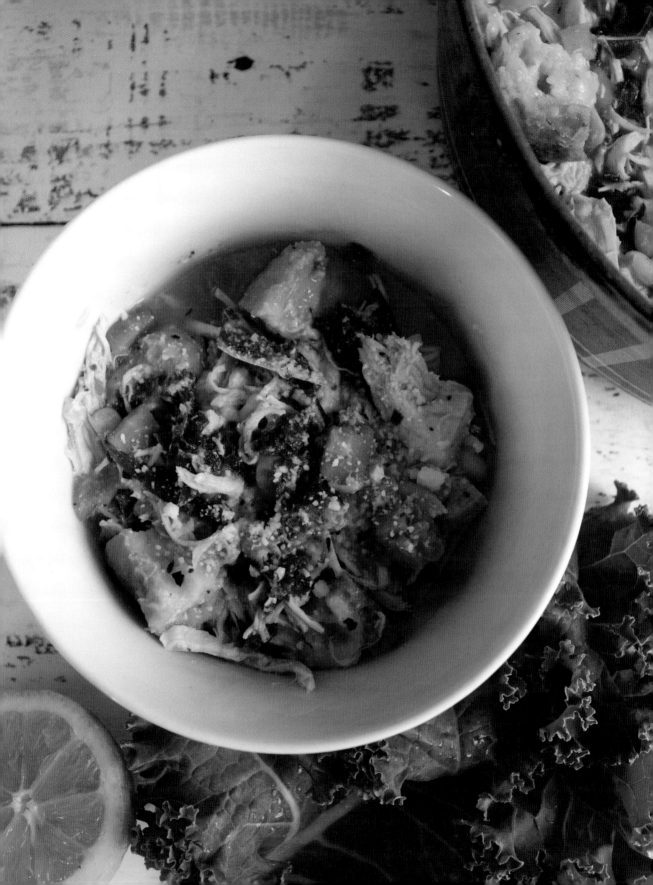

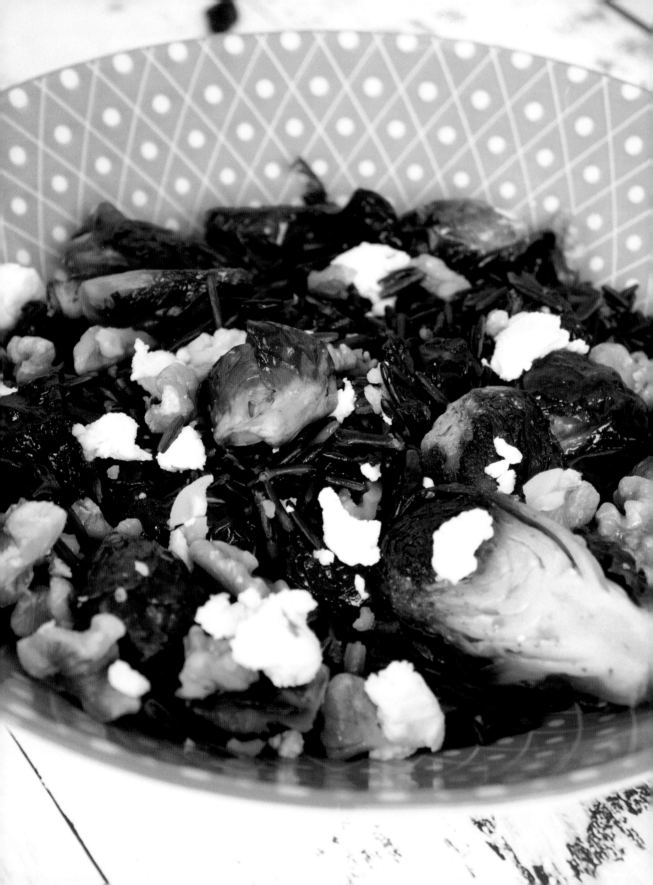

Warm Grain Bowl

The anatomy of a grain bowl consists of a well-cooked starch, roasted vegetables, protein (or dairy), and some flavorful toppings, and this recipe has all of those essentials. These grain bowls are a great vessel to pack in nutrition through roasted vegetables. Cruciferous vegetables in particular, such as cabbage, broccoli, kale, radishes, and Brussel sprouts, can be more bitter in flavor. Roasting allows for their flavor to shine and provides a rich source of fiber, folate, choline, and vitamin K.

Serves: 2 | Prep time: 15 minutes | Cook time: 20 minutes

INGREDIENTS

1 cup Brussels sprouts, sliced in half

2 tablespoons extra-virgin olive oil, divided

¼ teaspoon salt

¼ teaspoon pepper

2 cups cooked wild rice

¼ cup dried cherries

¼ cup walnuts

¼ cup goat cheese, crumbled

balsamic glaze, to serve (optional)

1. Preheat the oven to 400°F. On a medium baking sheet, add the sliced Brussels sprouts and top with 1 tablespoon of olive oil, salt, and pepper, tossing the ingredients together to ensure that each sprout is covered with oil.

2. Place the baking sheet in the oven and roast for 20 minutes, until the sprouts are tender and caramelized. Allow the vegetables to cool.

3. In a medium mixing bowl, combine the cooked wild rice, brussels sprouts, dried cherries, walnuts, and remaining tablespoon of olive oil. Toss all of the ingredients to combine.

4. Divide the grain mixture into 2 bowls and top each with crumbled goat cheese and balsamic glaze, if desired. The dish is best served warm.

#MomHack: The variations for this bowl are endless. Clean out the fridge or use leftovers, as you can swap in any grain or protein you have on hand. Swap out the toppings to include different dried fruits and nuts to experiment with various flavor profiles and add seasonal vegetables based on availability.

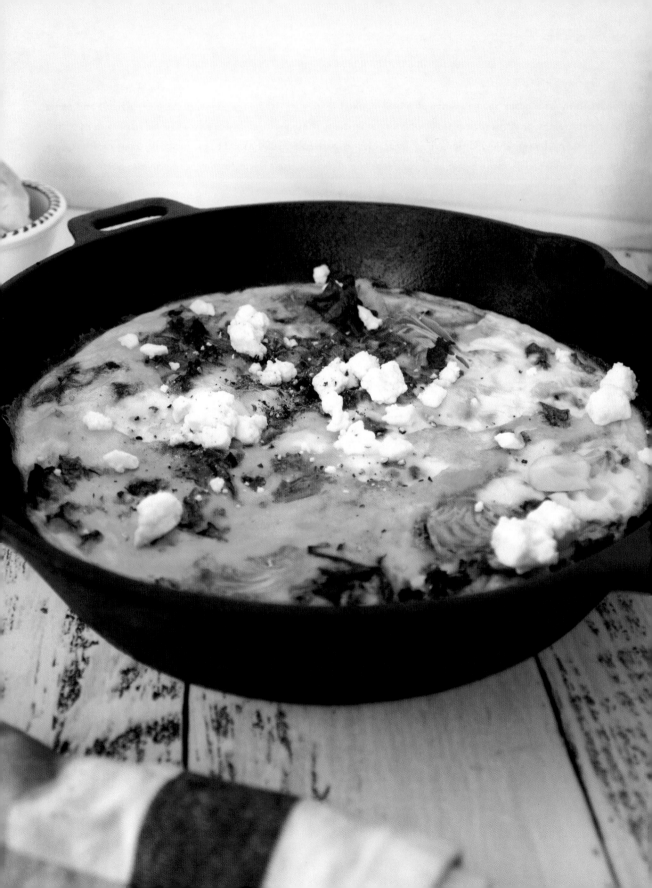

Mediterranean Frittata

Frittatas are known as the holy grail of versatile meals. They are simple to prepare, you can add just about whatever vegetables and ingredients you have on hand, and they are, of course, delicious. This recipe is packed with Mediterranean flavor and is rich in protein, fiber, calcium, and phytonutrients from colorful vegetables.

Serves: 8 | Prep time: 10 minutes | Cook time: 25 minutes

INGREDIENTS

1 tablespoon olive oil

2 cloves garlic, minced

1 bunch kale, chopped

salt and pepper, to taste

1 (14-ounce) can artichokes, drained

¼ cup sun-dried tomatoes, drained

8 eggs

¼ cup milk

¼ cup feta cheese crumbles, to serve

1. In a cast-iron skillet, heat the olive oil over medium heat. Preheat the oven to 400°F.

2. Add the minced garlic to the skillet and sauté for 2 minutes, until fragrant, then add the chopped kale and salt and pepper to taste.

3. Add the artichokes and sun-dried tomatoes to the skillet and sauté all of the vegetables until tender, about 5 minutes.

4. In a medium bowl, whisk the eggs together with the milk, then add them to skillet.

5. Lower the heat and allow the eggs to sit in the skillet until the edges begin to set, about 4 to 5 minutes (eggs should not be runny).

6. Using an oven mitt, move the skillet to the oven and bake for 8 to 10 minutes, until the eggs are set.

7. Remove the skillet from the oven and add feta cheese on top to serve.

#MomHack: Cooking ingredients in a cast-iron skillet can boost the iron content of your meals. While you certainly should aim to get iron through your diet (some is provided by the dark leafy greens in this recipe!), using a cast-iron skillet can support moms looking to boost their iron stores during postpartum.

Postpartum Power Bowl

Power bowls are essentially a fancier term for making leftovers into a nutrient-packed, delicious meal! A power bowls consists of a grain/starch, a protein, a sauce or dressing for dietary fat, and vegetables. This recipe has an Asian flair and is perfect for postpartum as it includes healing ginger, cruciferous vegetables rich in fiber and choline, and salmon rich in omega-3 fatty acids and iodine.

Serves: 2 | Prep time: 15 minutes | Cook time: 15 minutes

INGREDIENTS

2 (6-ounce) salmon fillets

1 teaspoon sea salt

1 teaspoon ground ginger

pepper, to taste

2 cups cooked brown rice

2 cups shredded cabbage

1 cup shelled edamame

1 medium avocado, pitted and sliced

FOR THE PEANUT SAUCE

½ cup creamy peanut butter

1 tablespoon honey

1 tablespoon soy sauce

1 teaspoon sriracha

2 cloves garlic

½ teaspoon ground ginger

½ cup water

juice of 1 lime

1. Preheat the oven to 400°F and spray a baking sheet with cooking spray, then set it aside.

2. Season the salmon fillets with salt, ginger, and pepper and place them on the prepared baking sheet. Bake in the oven for 15 minutes, until cooked throughout.

3. In each of 2 bowls, place 1 cup of rice, 1 cup of cabbage, ½ cup of edamame, and half of the avocado.

4. Place the salmon on top of each bowl.

5. To make the peanut sauce, add all of the ingredients to a blender and blend for 1 to 2 minutes until creamy.

6. Drizzle the desired amount of peanut sauce over each bowl.

#MomHack: You can repurpose leftovers of grains and proteins from dinners throughout the week by making differently themed power bowls. For example, try Greek with couscous, feta, and cucumbers, or Mexican with rice, black beans, cheese, and peppers, or simply pile on your grain, starch, and veggies and top with a sauce/dressing of your choice.

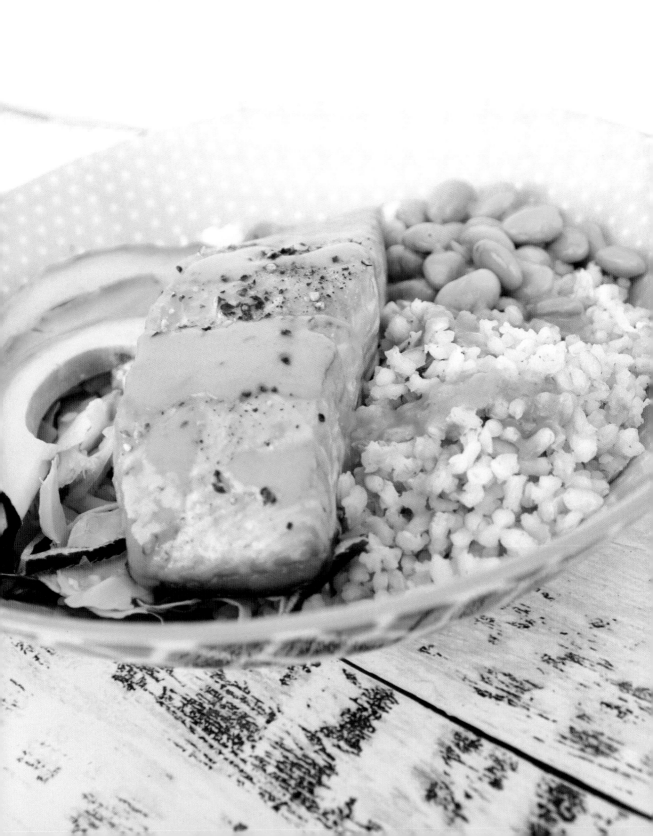

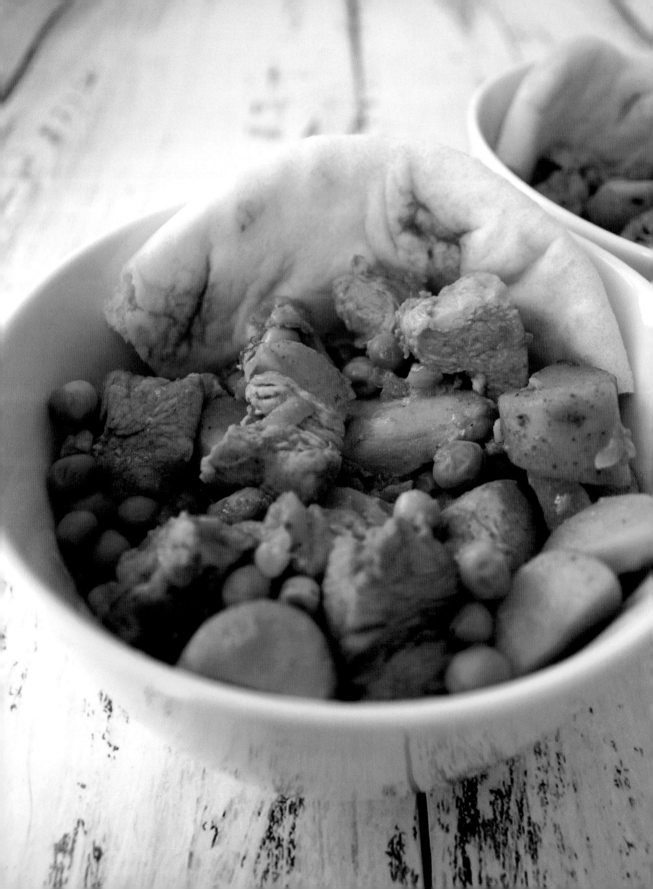

Quick Chicken Curry

While this recipe certainly does not do authentic curry justice, it does embody the classic flavors and comes together quickly. Not only is curry delicious and nourishing, it contains warming and antioxidant-rich spices that reduce inflammation and aid healing. The peas add brightness as well as provide a great source of folate and fiber to the dish.

Serves: 4 | Prep time: 15 minutes | Cook time: 25 minutes

INGREDIENTS

1 tablespoon olive oil

1 medium yellow onion, diced

2 to 3 cloves garlic, minced

1 pound boneless chicken breast or chicken thighs, diced

1 teaspoon ground ginger

3 tablespoons curry powder

1 teaspoon salt, plus more to taste

1 cup chicken stock

1 cup quartered Yukon gold potatoes

1 cup coconut milk

½ cup green peas

juice of 1 lime

fresh cilantro (optional)

cooked rice and naan bread, to serve

1. In a skillet over medium heat, heat the olive oil and add the diced onion and garlic. Sauté for 2 to 3 minutes, until fragrant.

2. Add the diced chicken to the skillet and sauté until browned, about 8 to10 minutes, until juices run clear. Then add the ginger, curry powder, and salt and stir to distribute the spices evenly over the chicken.

3. Continue cooking the chicken for 5 minutes to allow the spice mixture to cook.

4. Add the chicken stock and potatoes and bring the mixture to a boil, then bring to a simmer for 10 minutes.

5. Add the coconut milk to the mixture and stir in the green peas. Simmer for 2 to 3 minutes.

6. Squeeze the lime into the curry, top with cilantro, if desired, and serve warm with rice and naan.

#MomHack: Curry serves as a great base recipe to experiment with different proteins such as tofu, legumes, and varying vegetables.

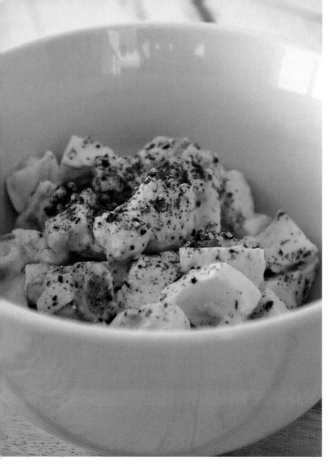

Avocado Egg Salad

This is not your average egg salad recipe! Creamy avocado adds the perfect texture as well as dietary fat, potassium, and fiber to this recipe. Paired with eggs for protein sustenance and a great source of choline, this salad is an easy way to build nutrient-dense snacks, so keep a batch on hand.

Serves: 2 to 3 | Prep time: 5 minutes | Cook time: None

INGREDIENTS

. . . .

4 hard-boiled eggs, diced

1 medium avocado, pitted and diced

½ tablespoon mayonnaise

1 teaspoon Dijon mustard

salt and pepper, to taste

. . . .

1. In a medium bowl, add the diced eggs, avocado, mayo, and mustard and stir to combine.

2. Add salt and pepper to taste and serve.

#MomHack: Serve the egg salad with crackers, in a wrap, or in a sandwich. To experiment with different flavors, you can swap out the mayonnaise with hummus, add in chopped fresh herbs such as dill or chives, or add in hot sauce or even curry powder to create your own variation.

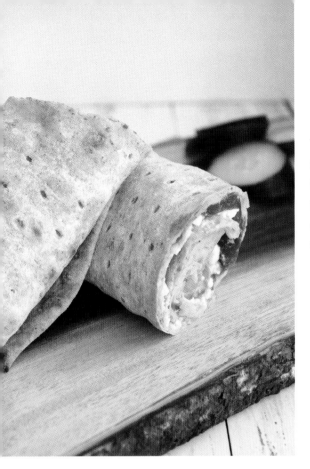

Roasted Salmon Wrap

This Mediterranean-inspired wrap is another delicious way to incorporate a dose of nutrient-rich salmon into your day. Not only does salmon provide the protein and omega-3 fatty acids needed during postpartum, it also provides an excellent source of B vitamins needed for tissue and blood cell production.

Serves: 2 | Prep time: 15 minutes | Cook time: 20 minutes

INGREDIENTS

2 (6-ounce) salmon fillets

salt and pepper, to taste

2 pieces lavash wraps

4 tablespoons hummus, divided

½ cup feta cheese crumbles

¼ cup roasted red pepper, drained

za'atar seasoning, to serve (optional)

1. Preheat the oven to 350°F and line a baking sheet with foil. Season the salmon with salt and pepper to taste. Bake the salmon for 20 minutes, until cooked thoroughly, and allow to cool.

2. Place the lavash wraps on a work surface and spread 2 tablespoons of hummus over the entire surface area of each wrap.

3. Place a salmon fillet in the center of each lavash and top with half of the feta and half of the red peppers. Top with za'atar seasoning, if desired.

4. Roll the wraps over the salmon fillet tightly so that all ingredients stay together cohesively.

5. Cut the wraps in half and serve.

#MomHack: Wraps can be prepared in a batch to snag from the fridge for a quick meal throughout the week. Mix and match ingredients in this recipe to create a flavor profile you enjoy! Wonderful additions would be sliced cucumber, olives, red onion, or spinach.

Shepherd's Pie with Instant Pot Mashed Potatoes

Shepherd's pie is a classic comfort food, and this recipe packs in nutrition for new moms. Ground beef provides a generous serving of protein for repairing muscle and tissues, as well as iron, zinc, and B vitamins for postpartum healing. Glutathione, an antioxidant that assists the body in fighting off free radicals that can damage cells, is found in high amounts in meat. Starch from the potatoes and fiber from the vegetables round this meal out to provide all of your needed macronutrients in one dish.

Serves: 10 | Prep time: 25 minutes | Cook time: 40 minutes

INGREDIENTS

1 tablespoon olive oil

1 pound ground beef (80/20 works best)

1 teaspoon garlic powder

½ teaspoon onion powder

1 teaspoon dried parsley

1 teaspoon salt

2 tablespoons tomato paste

1 teaspoon Worcestershire sauce

1 (10-ounce) bag frozen mixed vegetables, thawed

2 tablespoons flour

1 cup water

FOR THE POTATOES

2 cups water

3 medium russet potatoes, peeled, with some skin on, and quartered

1 tablespoon salted butter

¾ cup milk

salt and pepper, to taste

1. Preheat the oven to 400°F.

2. In an Instant Pot or pressure cooker, place the potatoes on high for 15 minutes.

3. While the potatoes cook, heat the olive oil over medium heat in a Dutch oven or ovenproof cookware.

4. Place the ground beef in the Dutch oven and, using a spatula, brown the ground beef and break it into smaller pieces, cooking it through, about 8 to 10 minutes.

5. Add the garlic powder, onion powder, dried parsley, salt, tomato paste, Worcestershire sauce, and mixed vegetables, and stir to combine.

6. Add the flour and stir to thicken the mixture, then add the water.

7. Allow the ground beef mixture to simmer for 2 to 3 minutes, then turn off the heat.

8. Once the potatoes have cooked for 15 minutes, do a quick release to complete cooking and add the potatoes to a medium mixing bowl to mash with the butter, milk, and salt and pepper to taste.

9. Scoop the prepared potatoes onto the meat mixture, spreading the potatoes with a spatula to distribute them over the top to cover the meat.

10. Place the Dutch oven in the oven for 20 to 25 minutes to cook. The pie is done when the potatoes are slightly browned on top. Serve warm.

#MomHack: This recipe's shortcuts reduce preparation time without skimping on flavor or nutrition. Frozen vegetables cook faster, garlic and onion powder pack in flavor without tedious chopping, and the potatoes are quick to cook in an Instant Pot or pressure cooker!

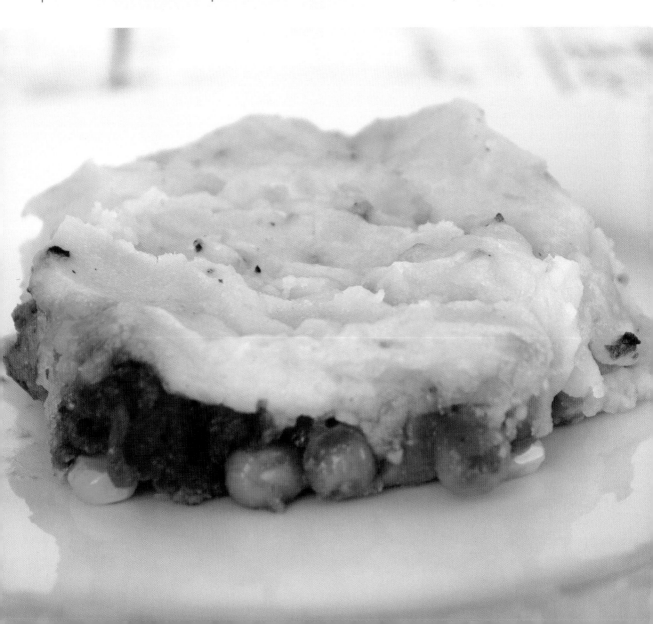

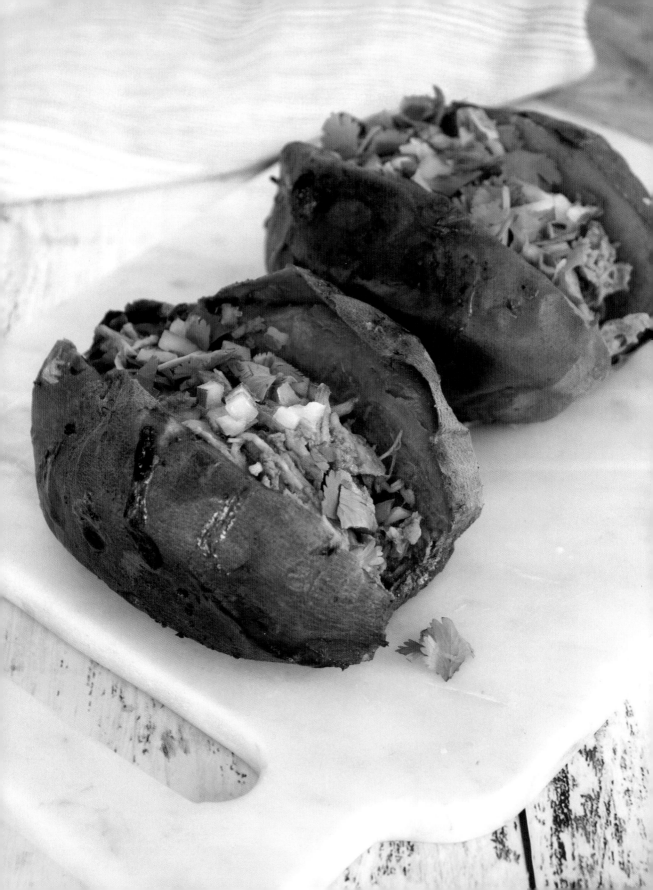

Pork Stuffed Sweet Potatoes

Shredded pork tenderloin is easy and tender when prepared in the slow cooker. It provides a great source of protein, iron, vitamins B6 and B-12, and magnesium. It is important to integrate a variety of meats (chicken, beef, fish, pork, lamb, etc.) and different cuts throughout postpartum, as different cuts can provide nutritional variety that serve to help restore and replenish after birth.

Serves: 4 to 6 | Prep time: 10 minutes |
Cook time: 45 minutes, plus 6 to 8 hours in slow cooker

INGREDIENTS

1 (16-ounce) pork tenderloin

½ cup barbecue sauce of choice, plus more to serve

4 medium sweet potatoes

1 tablespoon olive oil

1 teaspoon salt

1 teaspoon pepper

½ cup diced red onion

1 bunch cilantro

shredded cheese, to serve

1. Preheat the oven to 425°F.

2. Place the pork tenderloin in the middle of the slow cooker and top it with the barbecue sauce. Cook on low for 6 to 8 hours, until the meat is tender.

3. Remove the roast from the slow cooker and place it on a work surface. Using 2 forks, shred the meat into fine pieces, then set it aside.

4. Poke holes on the outside of the sweet potatoes with a fork.

5. Place the potatoes on a medium baking sheet and coat with the olive oil, salt, and pepper, covering all sides of the sweet potatoes.

6. Bake the sweet potatoes for 40 to 45 minutes until tender throughout, and allow them to cool.

7. Once the potatoes have cooled, slice them down the center to make a space for the pulled pork, and top each potato with ½ to ¾ cup of the pulled pork mixture.

8. Top with red onion, cilantro, cheese, and additional barbecue sauce and serve.

#MomHack: Slow cookers are a great way to cook proteins quickly. Be sure to cook this pork tenderloin on low (6 to 8 hours) as it ensures that the meat stays nice and tender!

Barbecue Tempeh Bowls

Tempeh is a wonderful addition to a postpartum staples list! Tempeh is made from fermented soybeans, which means it is rich in protein but also provides prebiotics (not to be confused with probiotics). Prebiotics are a type of fiber that promotes the growth of "good" bacteria in the gut and helps provide optimal digestion.

Serves: 2 | Prep time: 15 minutes | Cook time: 20 minutes

INGREDIENTS

1 (8-ounce) package tempeh, cut into small triangles

¼ cup barbecue sauce

2 bell peppers, red and yellow, cut into strips

½ small yellow onion, sliced

1 tablespoon olive oil

salt and pepper, to taste

2 cups pineapple spears, cut into cubes

2 cups cooked white rice, to serve

1 bunch green onions, diced, to serve

sesame seeds, to serve

1. Preheat the oven to 425°F and spray a large baking sheet with cooking spray.

2. Place the tempeh triangles on one third of the baking sheet and toss with the barbecue sauce, ensuring that each triangle is coated with sauce. Set it aside.

3. Place the peppers and onion on another third of the baking sheet and toss with the olive oil, salt, and pepper.

4. Place the pineapple on the remaining third of the baking sheet and place the sheet in the oven to cook for 20 minutes, until the peppers and onions are tender. Remove the pan from the oven to allow it to cool.

5. Plate the cooked rice in two bowls and top each with half of the tempeh, peppers, and pineapple.

6. Top each bowl with green onions and sesame seeds, as desired.

#MomHack: One pan and done for a simple and flavorful meal. If you need to cut down the prep time, you can purchase microwavable rice that cooks in 90 seconds.

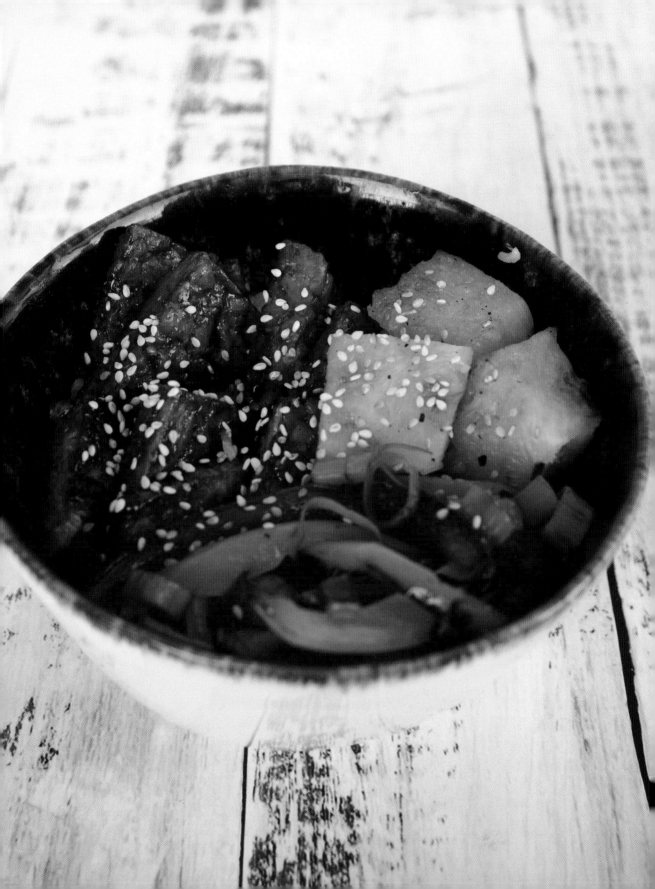

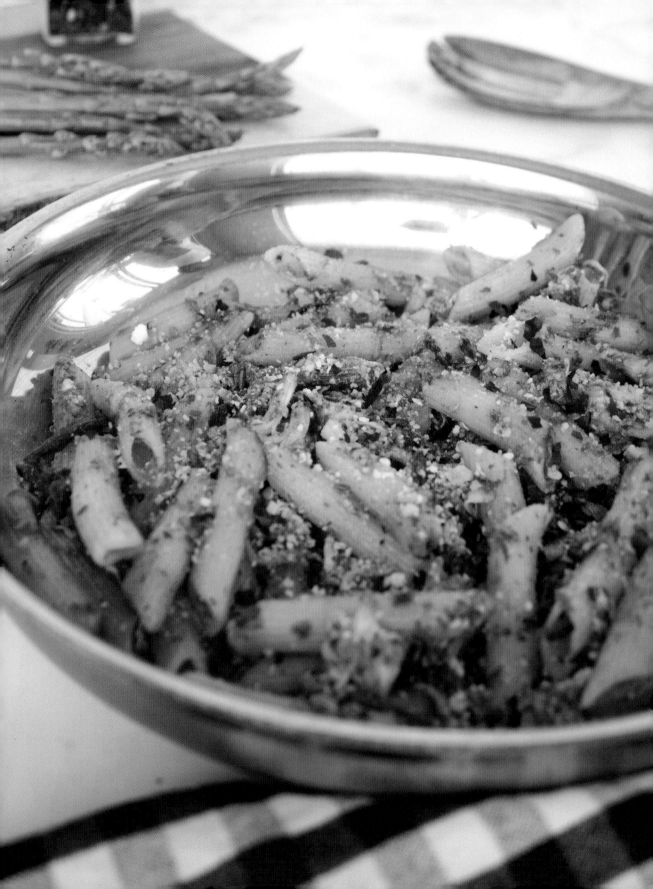

Pesto Chicken Pasta

Pasta is a classic comfort food fit for postpartum with the addition of colorful vegetables and flavorful pesto. Basil, which forms the foundation of pesto, provides the rich flavor and natural antioxidants in this dish, alongside lycopene-rich peppers and sun-dried tomatoes. Penne, ziti, or rigatoni would be good pasta choices.

Serves: 3 to 4 | Prep time: 15 minutes | Cook time: 15 minutes

INGREDIENTS

1 (8-ounce) package dry pasta

1 tablespoon olive oil

1 bunch asparagus, trimmed and cut into thirds

2 pieces roasted red peppers, sliced

2 tablespoons sun-dried tomatoes with oil

salt and pepper, to taste

⅓ cup prepared pesto (a jarred pesto or the Walnut Pesto on page 114 work great)

2 cups cooked chicken, shredded or cut into cubes

Parmesan cheese, to taste

red pepper flakes, to serve

1. Bring a saucepan filled with water to a boil, then add the pasta. Cook it for 8 to 10 minutes, until al dente (firm to touch).

2. While the pasta is cooking, prepare a medium skillet and heat the olive oil over medium heat. Add the asparagus and sauté for 3 to 4 minutes, until tender.

3. Add the red peppers, sun-dried tomatoes, and salt and pepper to taste and stir to combine so flavors can meld together.

4. Once the pasta is al dente, drain it and add the hot pasta to the skillet to combine.

5. Add the pesto to the skillet and stir to combine, then add the shredded chicken.

6. Top the skillet with Parmesan cheese and chili pepper flakes as desired, and serve.

#MomHack: Cook up a few extra chicken breasts to have on hand for sandwiches, wraps, and pastas. If you don't have any leftover chicken, you can purchase a plain rotisserie chicken and shred it with two forks to add to this dish.

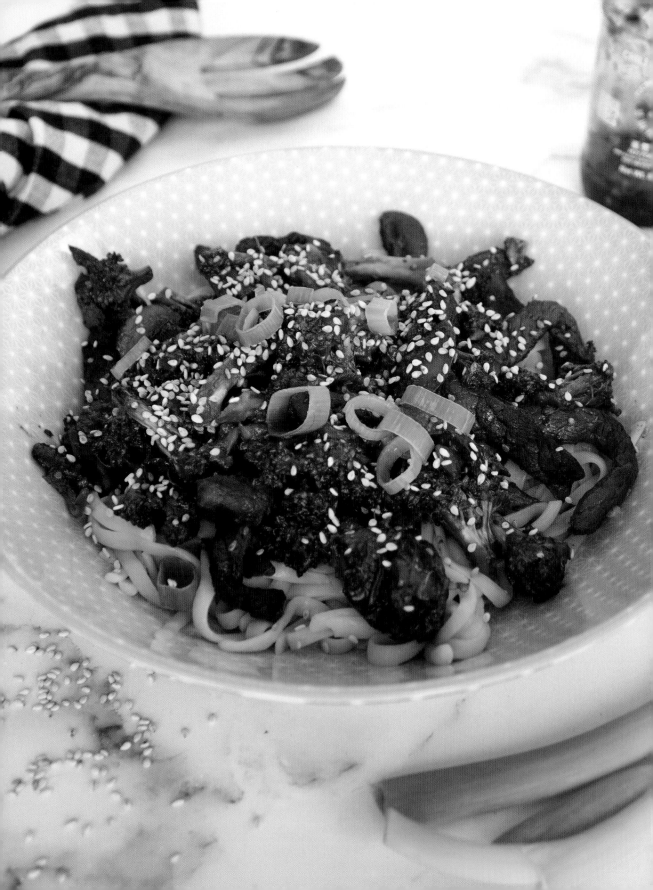

Stir-Fried Beef and Broccoli

Stir-fries make great lunch and dinner options for postpartum. The thin slices of beef cook quickly and provide a punch of iron, protein, and B vitamins—all integral nutrients during postpartum recovery.

Serves: 4 | Prep time: 10 minutes | Cook time: 15 to 20 minutes

INGREDIENTS

⅓ cup soy sauce

⅓ cup water

1 tablespoon honey

½ tablespoon brown sugar

1 tablespoon sesame seeds

1 teaspoon ground ginger

2 cloves garlic, minced

1 tablespoon cornstarch

2 tablespoons sesame oil, divided

2 cups broccoli florets

1 cup mushrooms, sliced

2 bunches green onions, sliced

1 pound flank steak stir-fry strips, sliced to ½-inch thickness

green onions, to serve (optional)

sesame seeds, to serve (optional)

1 package brown rice pad thai noodles, cooked, to serve

1. Prepare the stir-fry sauce by combining the soy sauce, water, honey, brown sugar, sesame seeds, ground ginger, garlic, and cornstarch in a small bowl. Whisk to combine, and set it aside.

2. In a medium skillet, heat 1 tablespoon of the sesame oil over medium heat and add the broccoli, mushrooms, and green onions, sautéing for 3 to 5 minutes until the vegetables are just tender. Remove them from the skillet and set them aside.

3. Add 1 tablespoon more of sesame oil to the skillet, followed by the steak strips. Cook for 6 to 8 minutes.

4. Add the vegetables back to the skillet with the prepared stir-fry sauce, stir to combine, and bring the mixture to a low simmer, 4 to 5 minutes, until the sauce has thickened.

5. Turn off the heat, top with additional green onions or sesame seeds, if desired, and serve over rice noodles.

#MomHack: Buying pre-chopped/sliced ingredients makes home-cooked, nutrient-dense meals possible during postpartum, when this time-consuming step might otherwise be a barrier to cooking. Most parents are willing to pay a bit more for these items to allow for the time savings in getting a warm, nutritious dinner on the table.

Sheet Pan Shrimp Bake

Shrimp serves as a tasty and quick source of protein and a great source of iodine, a nutrient you need for postpartum recovery. This one-pan meal contains all of the needed macronutrients, colorful vegetables, and fresh herbs, all of which amount to a meal rich in antioxidants and fiber.

Serves: 4 | Prep time: 15 minutes | Cook time: 18 to 20 minutes

INGREDIENTS

1 pound shrimp, peeled and deveined, with tails removed

3 cloves garlic, minced

2 tablespoons olive oil, divided

1 teaspoon salt

juice of 1 lemon

1 bunch basil, minced

pepper, to taste

2 zucchinis, sliced into 1-inch rounds, ends discarded

2 yellow squash, sliced into 1-inch rounds, ends discarded

½ pound baby red potatoes, quartered

red pepper flakes, to serve

1. Preheat the oven to 425°F and coat a medium baking sheet with cooking spray, then set it aside.

2. In a medium bowl, combine the shrimp, garlic, 1 tablespoon olive oil, salt, lemon, basil, and pepper, allowing the flavors to combine. Set it aside.

3. Place the zucchini and squash on the baking sheet.

4. Add the baby potatoes alongside the zucchini and squash, toss with an additional 1 tablespoon of olive oil, salt, and pepper, coating the vegetables and potatoes thoroughly.

5. Place the baking sheet with the potatoes and vegetables in the oven and bake for 10 minutes. When complete, remove the sheet from the oven, toss the vegetables, and add the shrimp to the baking sheet.

6. Bake for an additional 6 to 8 minutes until the shrimp is opaque and the potatoes are tender, remove it from the oven, and allow to cool. Serve.

#MomHack: One-pan meals make for easy cleanup. If you swap the shrimp out for a protein of your choice, adjust the cooking time accordingly as shrimp tends to cook more quickly in the oven, as opposed to chicken, beef, or other proteins.

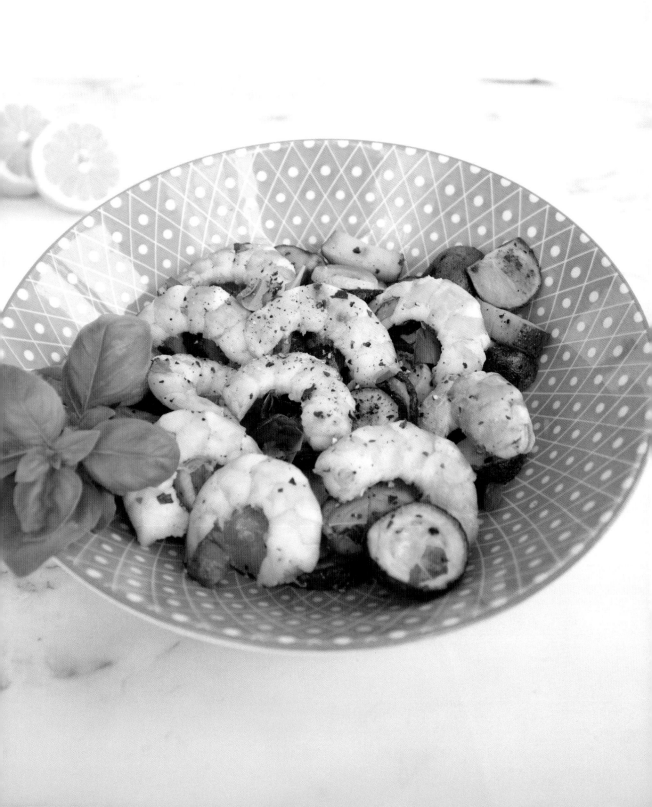

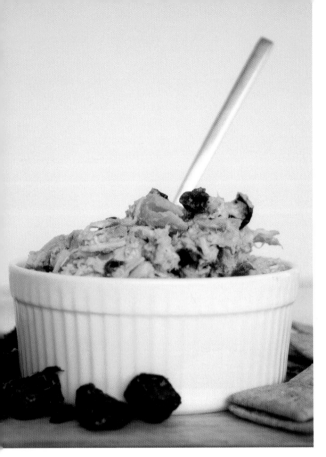

Curried Chicken Salad

Chicken salad gets a flavor boost with colorful curry powder in this recipe. Using spices such as curry powder, which contains a combination of turmeric, coriander, and chili powder, has been shown to have anti-inflammatory effects to aid in postpartum healing.

Serves: 4 | Prep time: 10 minutes | Cook time: None

INGREDIENTS

2 cups shredded chicken

2 tablespoons mayonnaise

¼ cup plain full-fat Greek yogurt

1 teaspoon curry powder, plus more to taste

¼ cup dried cranberries

¼ cup crumbled walnuts

1 stalk celery, thinly sliced

2 stalks green onion, thinly sliced

salt and pepper, to taste

1. In a medium bowl, add the chicken, mayonnaise, yogurt, and curry powder and stir to combine.

2. Add the remaining ingredients, seasoning with salt and pepper to taste. You can serve this salad immediately; however, it is best when chilled for 10 minutes in the refrigerator before serving.

#MomHack: A combination of mayonnaise and Greek yogurt provides the right amount of flavor and creaminess. However, feel free to increase one or the other based on your taste preference. Chicken salad makes a great base to sample different ingredients. Experiment with dried fruits such as golden raisins or cherries, nuts such as pecans or cashews, or vegetables such as shredded carrots or diced bell peppers for added crunch.

Chapter 8

Snacks & Sides

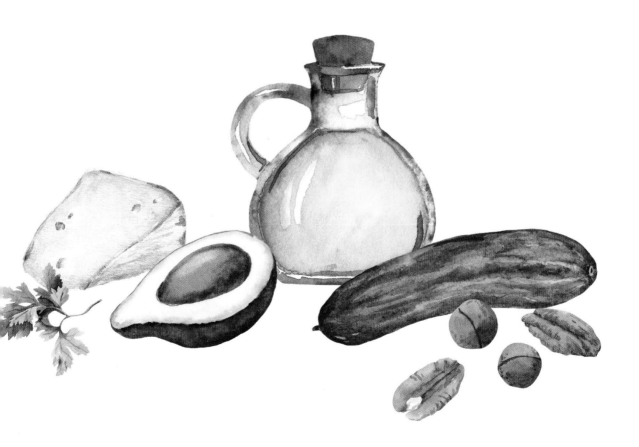

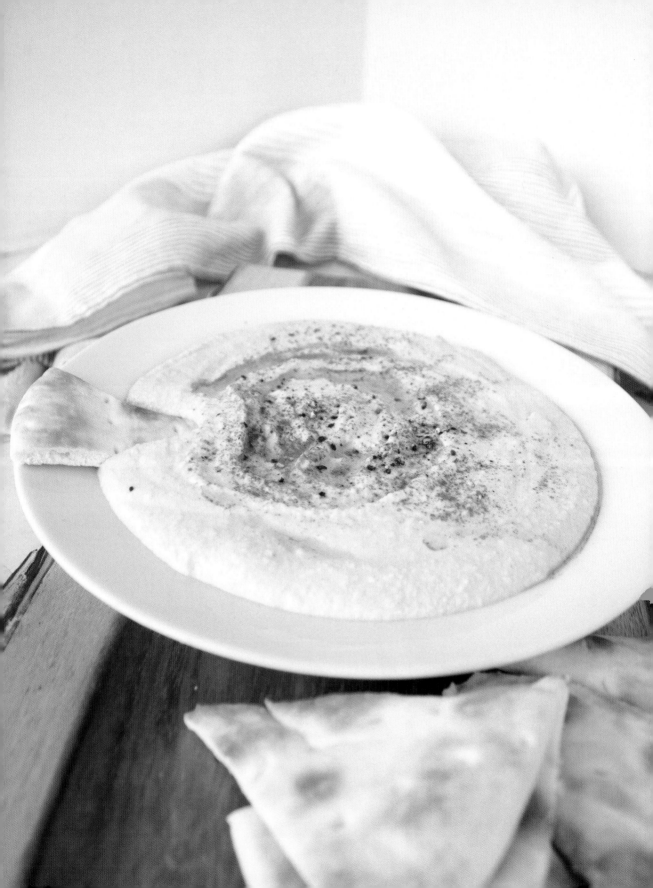

Garlic Hummus

Super-nutritious and packed with plant-based protein, this is a staple recipe that has all the essential ingredients. Tahini, a ground sesame paste, gives rich texture and savory flavor in addition to providing a good source of copper and selenium.

Serves: 8 | Prep time: 5 minutes | Cook time: None

INGREDIENTS

⅓ cup tahini

3 tablespoons cold water, plus more as needed

2 tablespoons extra-virgin olive oil

4 cloves garlic, peeled

½ teaspoon ground cumin

½ teaspoon sea salt, plus more to taste

juice of 1 lemon, plus more to taste

1 (15-ounce) can garbanzo beans, rinsed and drained

1. In a food processor, combine the tahini, water, olive oil, garlic, cumin, sea salt, and lemon juice. Puree the ingredients until the mixture combines and reaches a smooth texture.

2. Add the garbanzo beans to the mixture and puree for 2 to 3 minutes, pausing intermittently to scrape down the sides of the food processor.

3. Test the mixture for thickness, adding more water if needed to reach a smooth texture.

4. Scrape the mixture out of the bowl and taste, adding more salt or lemon juice as desired.

5. Store in the refrigerator for 3 days in an airtight container.

#MomHack: For moms who are healing from birth and facing a ravenous appetite, hummus is a great option to boost nutrition in a variety of meals. Slather it onto crackers or fresh-cut vegetables, or add it onto a sandwich or wrap.

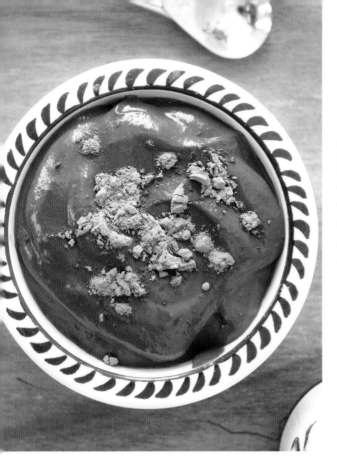

Chocolate Avocado Pudding

Of course, you can have regular pudding, but why have regular pudding when you can have both flavor and amazing nutrition? I've created different forms of chocolate pudding over the years, but I have found this basic recipe provides the best results. Most people are shocked to find that the velvety and smooth texture of this recipe comes from avocados!

Serves: 4 | Prep time: 5 minutes | Cook time: None

INGREDIENTS

2 ripe medium avocados, pitted and diced, with skin removed

½ cup cocoa powder

¼ cup honey or sweetener of choice, such as maple syrup

3 tablespoons milk of choice

pinch of sea salt

shredded coconut, to top (optional)

1. Place the avocados in a food processor or blender.

2. Add all of the remaining ingredients and process until combined and smooth. Scrape down the sides of the bowl as needed.

3. Transfer the mixture to a bowl to refrigerate for 30 to 40 minutes.

4. Spoon into 4 small bowls for serving and top with coconut as desired.

#MomHack: Experiment with this base recipe and adjust the sweetener to your liking, as well as using different toppings as desired, such as nuts, coconut, and fruit. You can also freeze the pudding if you'd like a creamier texture.

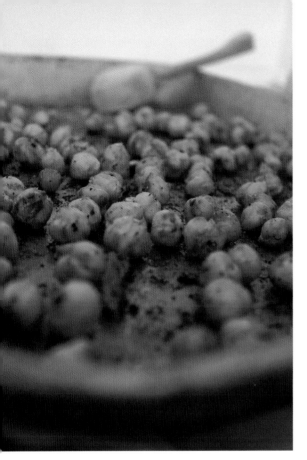

Roasted Garbanzo Beans

The ever-versatile garbanzo bean is tossed with olive oil and spices, and roasted to crunchy perfection to make a savory snack in this recipe. There are many variations of this recipe and many yet to be uncovered, so feel free to experiment with different spices. But I am partial to the inclusion of garlic and paprika as they add flavor and warmth.

Serves: 4 | Prep time: 5 minutes |
Cook time: 25 minutes

INGREDIENTS

1 (14-ounce) can garbanzo beans, rinsed and drained

1 tablespoon extra-virgin olive oil

1 teaspoon garlic powder

½ teaspoon salt

pinch of paprika, plus more to taste

pepper, to taste

cayenne pepper, to taste

1. Preheat the oven to 400°F. In a bowl, combine the garbanzo beans, olive oil, and spices and ensure that all the beans are coated well.

2. Distribute the garbanzo beans evenly on a baking sheet and place it in the oven.

3. About halfway through the baking time (about 12 minutes), stir the garbanzo beans to ensure that they roast on all sides, and continue baking for the remainder of the time until they are dry and crispy on the outside.

4. Remove the garbanzo beans from the oven and let them cool. Garbanzo beans can be served warm or cool and stored in a sealed container in the fridge.

#MomHack: These garbanzo beans not only make a wonderful snack to munch on in between meals but also work great as a way to elevate salads, bowls, and soups.

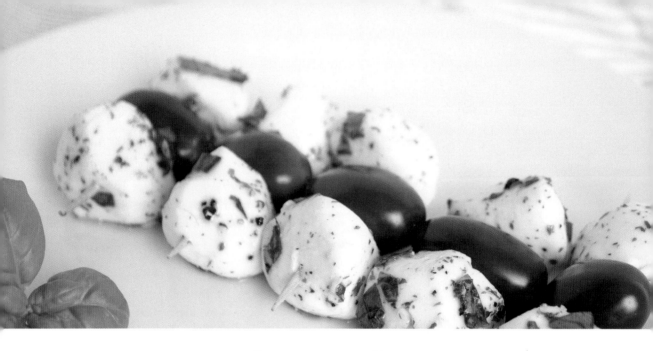

Caprese Bites

Simple ingredients provide maximum flavor in this quick and easy snack. Keeping an assortment of cheeses in the fridge, such as cherry-sized mozzarella used in this recipe, makes for an easy way to add flavor, protein, and calcium to meals and snacks.

Serves: 2 to 4 | Prep time: 5 minutes | Cook time: None

INGREDIENTS

1 (8-ounce) container cherry mozzarella

1 pint cherry tomatoes

1 bunch fresh basil, torn into small pieces

1 teaspoon extra-virgin olive oil

salt and pepper, to taste

balsamic glaze, to taste

1. Combine the mozzarella, tomatoes, basil, and oil in a medium bowl and toss to combine. Add salt and pepper to taste.

2. Skewer 1 tomato and 2 pieces of mozzarella on a toothpick.

3. Top with balsamic glaze, if desired, and serve.

#MomHack: Make a batch to snack on throughout the week and use the remainder to toss into the Caprese Pasta Salad (page 61). Or serve alongside chicken, or add ingredients like olives or roasted vegetables to the skewer.

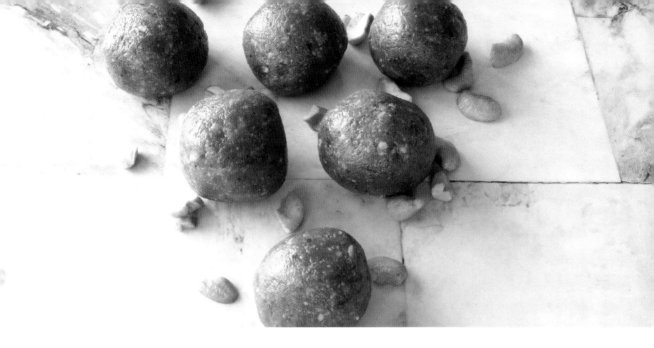

Cashew Date Bites

Dates promote optimal postnatal digestive health by providing both soluble and insoluble fiber. Dates are also a rich source of magnesium and protect against oxidative stress to nourish depleted tissues after birth.

Serves: 4 | Prep time: 2 minutes | Cook time: None

INGREDIENTS

1 cup pitted Medjool dates

1 cup cashews

coconut flakes, to top

chia seeds, to top

1. Place the dates and nuts in a food processor. Pulse for 1 to 2 minutes, until the mixture forms into a large ball.

2. Scoop 2 tablespoons of the mixture and roll it with your hands to combine into a ball. Repeat with the remaining mixture. Top with coconut flakes and chia seeds, as desired.

3. Place in fridge for about 5 minutes to allow bites to firm up. Store in the fridge for up to 5 days.

#MomHack: These bites come together in a food processor in 2 minutes flat. Have a batch on hand for quick and nutrient-dense snacks you can enjoy during marathon nursing sessions or in the stretches between meals. You can swap the cashews for any nut of choice. I have found that cashews tend to help the ball hold its shape and provide a rich, nutty flavor.

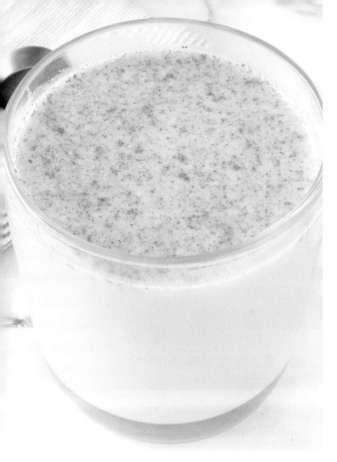

Golden Milk

Nutritionally, turmeric is touted for its cancer-fighting antioxidants and anti-inflammatory properties. Evidence shows it is beneficial in fighting diabetes, cancer, Crohn's disease, and other chronic diseases. Golden Milk is a great way to incorporate this spice. In Ayurvedic medicine, mothers are served Golden Milk before bedtime to assist with the absorption of powerful anti-inflammatory qualities. This recipe pairs the active ingredient in turmeric, curcumin, with black pepper, which assists in boosting the absorption of turmeric in the body.

Serves: 4 | Prep time: 2 minutes |
Cook time: 20 minutes

INGREDIENTS

4 cups milk of choice

2 tablespoons honey, plus more to taste

2 teaspoons ground turmeric

2 teaspoons ground cinnamon, plus more to taste

dash of ground cardamom

dash of pepper

1. Combine all of the ingredients in a small saucepan set on low heat. Heat for 20 minutes to let the flavors simmer and combine, gently whisking as needed.

2. Ladle the milk into cups and top it with ground cinnamon and additional honey for more sweetness.

#MomHack: To include turmeric in your diet, add it to the cooking water when preparing grains such as brown rice and quinoa, as well as to any dishes that maintain an earthy, warm taste, such as lentils and stews.

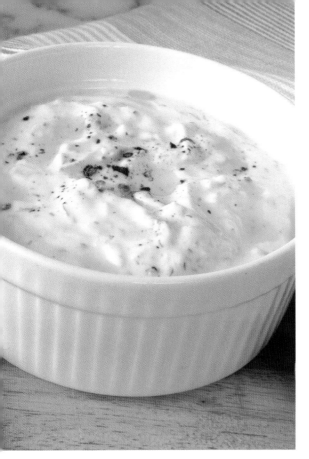

Tzatziki Sauce

This simple and refreshing Greek yogurt sauce can be piled on top of grilled meats, alongside roasted vegetables, or served with warm pita bread. Fresh herbs, garlic, and olive oil add flavor and a healthy dose of anti-inflammatory properties. Boasting a dose of protein and calcium, it makes a perfect postpartum staple to keep on hand.

Serves: 8 | Prep time: 10 minutes |
Cook time: None

INGREDIENTS

1 cucumber, peeled and shredded

2 cups plain full-fat Greek yogurt

2 to 3 cloves garlic, minced

2 tablespoons olive oil

1 bunch fresh dill, chopped

1 teaspoons salt

pepper, to taste

squeeze of fresh lemon

1. Place the shredded cucumber in a strainer to drain the water. Alternatively, you can squeeze the shreds over the sink to reduce the liquid.

2. Combine the yogurt, garlic, and olive oil in a bowl and stir to combine.

3. Add the shredded cucumber once it is completely drained.

4. Add the dill to the yogurt mixture with the salt, pepper, and lemon, to taste.

#MomHack: Tzatziki can be made in a large batch and kept in the fridge for 4 days. Pile it up in a snack bowl alongside hummus and fresh vegetables, for a high-fiber postpartum snack you can scoop up with crackers.

Apricot Almond Granola

Apricots and almonds are a dynamic duo in this super-simple granola recipe. Apricots add a brightness and texture and a healthy dose of soluble fiber to help feed your gut microbiome. Dried fruits normally get a bad reputation; however, they make a quick and dense postpartum snack to help keep blood sugar levels even.

Makes: 6 (½-cup) servings | Prep time: 10 minutes | Cook time: 30 to 40 minutes

INGREDIENTS

3 cups rolled oats

1 cup almonds

¾ cup chopped dried apricots

¼ cup ground flaxseeds

½ teaspoon salt

1 teaspoon ground cinnamon

1 teaspoon ground cardamom

½ cup honey

2 tablespoons coconut oil, melted

1 teaspoon vanilla or almond extract

1 egg white

1. Line a large baking sheet with parchment paper and preheat the oven to 300°F.

2. In a large bowl, combine the oats, almonds, apricots, flaxseeds, salt, cinnamon, and cardamom.

3. Pour in the honey, coconut oil, and extract and stir to combine to ensure that all oats get coated.

4. Whisk the egg white in a small bowl and add it to the oat mixture, stirring to combine thoroughly.

5. Spread the mixture on the lined baking sheet and bake for 15 to 20 minutes.

6. Remove the granola from the oven. Using a spatula, gently flip sections of the granola (this creates chunks in the mixture) and bake for another 15 to 20 minutes, until the granola mixture is dry to the touch.

7. Remove the granola from the oven and let the mixture cool, breaking the granola into pieces of desired size.

#MomHack: Store the granola in an airtight container or mason jar and layer it on top of protein-rich Greek yogurt with berries, or keep a jar on hand to munch on clusters when a snack craving hits.

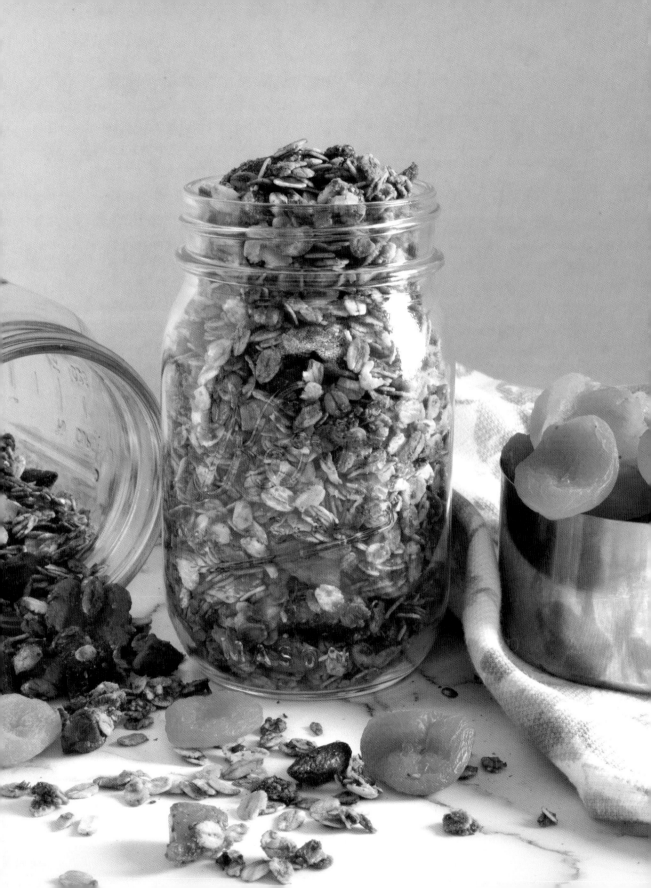

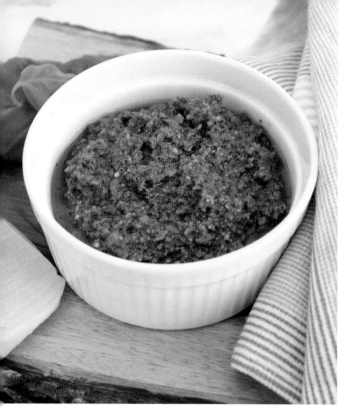

Walnut Pesto

This pesto takes a different turn from the usual pine nuts. Walnuts are energy dense, given their high fat content, and are packed with vitamins and minerals such as folic acid, copper, and vitamin E.

Serves: 10 | Prep time: 10 minutes |
Cook time: None

INGREDIENTS

. . . .

¼ cup walnuts

½ cup Parmigiano Reggiano cheese

3 cloves garlic

2 cups basil leaves

¼ cup extra-virgin olive oil

¼ teaspoon salt

. . . .

1. In a food processor, combine the walnuts, cheese, and garlic, pulsing for 20 to 30 seconds, until the walnuts form a paste.

2. Add the basil to the processor and continue to process the mixture, gradually adding olive oil and salt to the bowl.

3. Scrape the sides of the bowl and continue to process, adding more olive oil if desired, until the mixture if thoroughly combined.

#MomHack: Pesto is a great way to add a flavor and nutrient boost to your favorite meals. Add a scoop on top of salmon or chicken, scramble it into eggs, or use it as a dip with vegetables. Pesto can be prepared in a larger batch, then frozen in an ice cube tray and thawed out to use when desired.

Chia Pudding

Chia seeds are small in size but mighty with nutrition! Just 2 tablespoons of these tiny little seeds contain a generous dose of fiber, protein, and fat. Chia seeds are also high in calcium, phosphorus, magnesium, and potassium (a very similar profile to dairy products), so in conjunction with milk, they provide a great boost for bone health!

Serves: 2 | Prep time: 8 to 10 minutes, plus 1 hour up to overnight to chill | Cook time: None

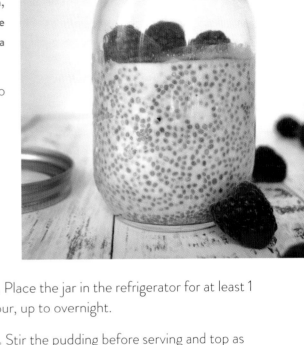

INGREDIENTS

1 cup milk of choice

4 tablespoons chia seeds

½ teaspoon vanilla extract

fresh diced fruit, sliced nuts, coconut, to top

1. Combine the milk, chia seeds, and vanilla extract in a jar and stir to combine.

2. Allow the mixture to sit for 8 to 10 minutes as the seeds start to gel, creating a thicker texture. Seal with an airtight lid.

3. Place the jar in the refrigerator for at least 1 hour, up to overnight.

4. Stir the pudding before serving and top as desired.

#MomhHack: Mix and match any toppings to use with this basic recipe. If you prefer a sweeter taste, try adding maple syrup or honey to the mix. You can include chia seeds in other ways throughout your diet. Use it as a topping for yogurt, on oatmeal, in smoothies, or even on salads.

Roasted Beets and Walnuts

Beets, a ruby-colored root vegetable, are packed with essential nutrients and flavor. Roasted beets often show up in salads or pickled. Nutritionally, the rich color of beets tells us that the vegetable is loaded with antioxidants, vitamins, and minerals. They are specifically high in potassium, iron, and vitamin C, as well as fiber. This side dish has simple yet pronounced flavors, pairing the beets with walnuts and fresh citrus. It can be eaten as a simple side to main courses, topped on salads, or simply enjoyed on its own.

Serves: 3 to 4 | Prep time: 10 minutes | Cook time: 25 minutes

INGREDIENTS

3 medium beets, greens removed, peeled, and diced into bite-size pieces.

1 tablespoon olive oil

1 teaspoon salt

¼ teaspoon pepper

1 medium orange, peeled into sections

½ cup walnuts

¼ cup feta crumbles

balsamic glaze, to serve

mint leaves, to serve

1. Preheat the oven to 425°F and spray a baking sheet with cooking spray.

2. In a medium bowl, toss the beets with olive oil, salt, and pepper

3. Place the beets on the baking sheet and bake for 25 minutes, until they are fork tender.

4. Allow the beets to cool.

5. In a medium bowl, combine the beets, orange sections, walnuts, and feta crumbles, and toss to combine.

6. Top with balsamic glaze and mint leaves as desired.

#MomHack: Roasting beets at home can be a production but adds to the flavor of this side. To avoid staining prepware, place plastic wrap on your cutting surface. If you want to avoid this step altogether or need to save on time, you can find beets already peeled and cooked at many grocery stores.

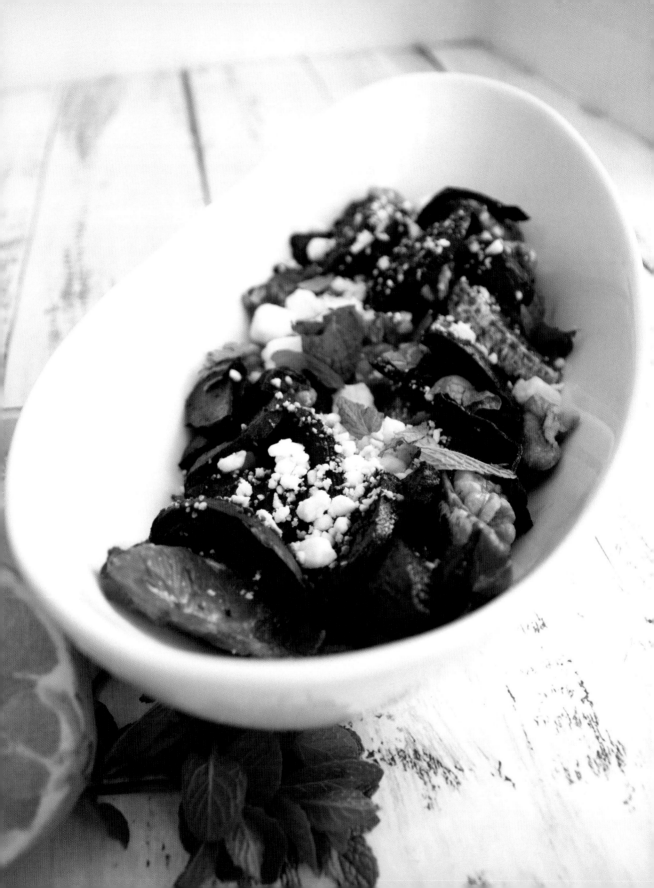

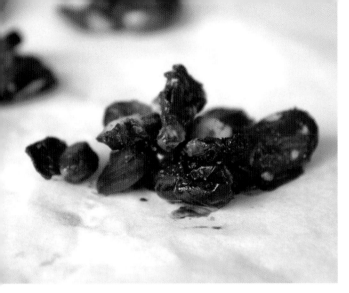

Chocolate Nut Clusters

These nut clusters provide the best of both sweet and salty flavors plus nutrition and satisfaction. Nuts provide protein and fat to help stabilize blood sugar throughout the day and also contain polyphenols, antioxidants that aid in the body's repair work.

Serves: 6 | Prep time: 15 minutes |
Cook time: 10 minutes, plus 20 minutes to chill

INGREDIENTS

2 cups unsalted mixed nuts, larger nuts loosely chopped (any variety)

½ cup dried cherries

½ to ¾ cup dark chocolate chips

1 tablespoon coconut oil, melted

1 teaspoon sea salt, as desired

1. Set the oven broiler on low.

2. Place the mixed nuts on a baking sheet and broil for 4 to 6 minutes, turning them often to ensure that they are toasting without burning.

3. Remove the baking sheet from the oven and allow the nuts to cool slightly. Once they are cooled, mix in the cherries.

4. To a microwave-safe bowl, add the melted coconut oil and the chocolate chips, using more if you prefer a sweeter cluster, and microwave in 30-second intervals, stirring the mixture after each interval, until a liquid forms.

5. Place the nut and cherry mixture in close proximity on a piece of parchment paper spread out on a work surface. Evenly drizzle the melted chocolate over the nuts and cherries, and sprinkle with sea salt as desired.

6. Place the mixture in the fridge to allow the clusters to bind together, about 20 minutes.

7. Remove the mixture from the fridge once clusters have formed, and break them into the desired size. Store them in the refrigerator in a sealed container.

#MomHack: Roasting seems like a silly step. However, it really is essential to boost the flavor! Keep a jar of these in the fridge for quick-and-satisfying snacking throughout the day. You will get a dose of protein and fiber and satisfy your desire for sweet and salty.

Cookie Dough Bites

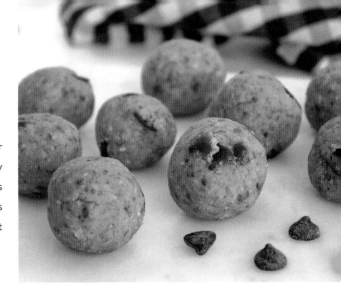

These bites are a quick, easy way to satisfy your sweet cravings while still serving up nutrition to carry you through the day! It seems as if cookie dough is everywhere in different forms, but I like this recipe as it integrates protein, fat, and carbohydrates to support regulated blood sugar.

Serves: 4 to 6, makes 12 to 14 balls |
Prep time: 5 minutes, plus 10 minutes to chill |
Cook time: None

INGREDIENTS

1 cup oat flour, finely ground

2 tablespoons ground flaxseeds

½ cup protein powder

½ cup smooth peanut butter (or nut butter of choice)

1 tablespoon coconut oil, melted

2 to 3 tablespoons milk of choice

⅓ cup dark chocolate chips

1. In a mixing bowl, combine the oat flour, flaxseeds, and protein powder. Set it aside.

2. Combine the peanut butter and coconut oil in a microwave-safe bowl and microwave in 20-second intervals until melted.

3. Pour the peanut butter and coconut oil into the mixing bowl with the oat flour mixture and stir to combine. Add the milk one tablespoon at a time to decrease the thickness of the mixture until all ingredients combine easily.

4. Once all of the ingredients have been combined, stir in the chocolate chips.

5. Using a cookie scoop, scoop about 2 tablespoons of the mixture and roll it between the palms of your hands to form a ball. Repeat with the remainder of the mixture.

6. Place the balls in a glass container for storage in the refrigerator, chilling them for 10 minutes to firm up.

#MomHack: No need to purchase oat flour; you can make your own using regular rolled oats by using a blender or food processor and pulsing a few times until the oats are a fine powder. Feel free to experiment with different ingredients, such as dried fruits, nuts, and seeds.

Stuffed Dates

Dried fruits such as dates provide concentrated energy for sleep-deprived moms. Pair the Medjool dates with savory tahini to provide fat, which assists in keeping blood sugar stable for sustained energy through the day.

Serves: 4 to 5 | Prep time: 5 minutes | Cook time: None

INGREDIENTS

10 whole Medjool dates

½ to ¾ cup tahini

2 to 3 tablespoons shredded coconut, to top

1. To pit the dates, slice them down center, remove the pit, and gently press open the sides of the dates to make room for the filling.

2. Scoop about 1 tablespoon of tahini per date and fill the date with it. Plate and top with shredded coconut. Serve immediately or store in an airtight container in the fridge.

#MomHack: Dried fruits are a great pantry staple to have on hand as a snack or to add flavor, texture, and color to salads and grain dishes.

Black Bean Dip

This dip makes for an easy snack throughout the day. The main staple of this dip, black beans, provide creamy texture and plant-based protein, fiber, and folate. Fresh cilantro, garlic, and red peppers provide an antioxidant boost.

Serves: 4 to 6 | Prep time: 5 minutes | Cook time: None

INGREDIENTS

1 (15-ounce) can black beans, drained

3 cloves garlic

2 pieces jarred roasted red peppers

1 bunch cilantro, stems removed

1 teaspoon ground cumin

dash of chili powder

juice of 1 lime

1. Combine all of the ingredients in a food processor or blender and pulse for 30 seconds to 1 minute, until the mixture is combined and reaches the desired thickness (dip should be thick and creamy with some small chunks of beans remaining).

#MomHack: Make this dip in a large batch and scoop it up with chopped vegetables or corn tortilla chips for a midday boost.

Conversions

VOLUME

U.S.	U.S. Equivalent	Metric
1 tablespoon (3 teaspoons)	½ fluid ounce	15 milliliters
¼ cup	2 fluid ounces	60 milliliters
⅓ cup	3 fluid ounces	90 milliliters
½ cup	4 fluid ounces	120 milliliters
⅔ cup	5 fluid ounces	150 milliliters
¾ cup	6 fluid ounces	180 milliliters
1 cup	8 fluid ounces	240 milliliters
2 cups	16 fluid ounces	480 milliliters

WEIGHT

U.S.	Metric
½ ounce	15 grams
1 ounce	30 grams
2 ounces	60 grams
¼ pound	115 grams
⅓ pound	150 grams
½ pound	225 grams
¾ pound	350 grams
1 pound	450 grams

TEMPERATURE

Fahrenheit (°F)	Celsius (°C)
140°F	60°C
150°F	65°C
160°F	70°C
170°F	75°C
300°F	150°C
325°F	165°C
350°F	175°C
375°F	190°C
400°F	200°C
425°F	220°C
450°F	230°C

Recommended Resources

4th Trimester Bodies Project
www.4thtrimesterbodiesproject.com
A collection of photography aimed at capturing the postpartum journey for all.

Health at Every Size
www.haescommunity.org
Information to cultivate compassion for all body sizes.

International Lactation Consultant Association
www.ilca.org
Resources for locating an International Board-Certified Lactation Consultant (IBCLC).

Intuitive Eating
www.intuitiveeating.org
Information on intuitive eating.

Postpartum Health Alliance
www.postpartumhealthalliance.org
Resources for postpartum mood and anxiety disorders; referrals for perinatal mental health professionals in the community.

Notes

1   Gwen Stern and Laurence Kruckman, "Multi-Disciplinary Perspectives on Post-Partum Depression: An Anthropological Critique," *Social Science Medicine* 17, no. 15 (1983): 1027–1041. doi:10.1016/0277-9536(83)90408-2.

2   M. Withers, N. Kharazmi, and E. Lim, "Traditional Beliefs and Practices in Pregnancy, Childbirth and Postpartum: A Review of the Evidence from Asian Countries," *Midwifery* 56 (January 2018): 158–170. doi:10.1016/j.midw.2017.10.019.

3   A. Conde, A. Rosas-Bermudez, F. Castano, and M. Norton, "Effects of Birth Spacing on Maternal, Perinatal, Infant, and Child Health: A Systematic Review of Causal Mechanisms," *Studies in Family Planning* 43, no 2. (June 2012): 93–114.

4   K. G. Dewey and R. J. Cohen, "Does Birth Spacing Affect Maternal or Child Nutritional Status? A Systematic Literature Review," *Maternal and Child Nutrition* 3, no. 3 (2007):151–173. doi: 10.1111/j.1740-8709.2007.00092.x.

5   M. E. Lovering, R. F. Rodgers, J. E. George, and D. L. Franko, "Exploring the Tripartite Influence Model of Body Dissatisfaction in Postpartum Women," *Body Image* 24 (2018): 44–54. doi:10.1016/j.bodyim.2017.12.001.

6   C. Dennis, K. Fung, S. Grigoriadis, G. Robinson, et al., "Traditional Postpartum Practices and Rituals: A Qualitative Systematic Review," *Women's Health 3,* no. 4 (July 2007): 487–502. doi. org/10.2217/17455057.3.4.487.

7   J. L. Pawluski, M. Li, and J. S. Lonstein, "Serotonin and Motherhood: From Molecules to Mood," *Front Neuroendocrinology* 53, (2019):100742. doi: 10.1016/j.yfrne.2019.03.001.

8   G. Sebastiani, A. Herranz Barbero, C. Borrás-Novell, et al., "The Effects of Vegetarian and Vegan Diet during Pregnancy on the Health of Mothers and Offspring," *Nutrients* 11, no. 3 (2019):557. doi: 10.3390/nu11030557.

9   F. M. Sacks, A. H. Lichtenstein, J. H. Y. Wu, et al., "Dietary Fats and Cardiovascular Disease: A Presidential Advisory from the American Heart Association," *Circulation* 136, no. 10 (2017): 1–23. doi:10.1161/CIR.0000000000000510.

10   E. K. Pawels and D. Volterrani, "Fatty Acid Facts, Part I. Essential Fatty Acids as Treatment for Depression, or Food for Mood?" *Drug News Perspectives* 21, no. 8 (2008):446–451. doi: 10.1358/ dnp.2008.21.8.1272136.

11   National Institutes of Health, "Nutrient Recommendations: Dietary Reference Intake (DRI)," https:// ods.od.nih.gov/Health_Information/Dietary_Reference_Intakes.aspx.

12   M. Azami, G. Badfar, Z. Khalighi, et al., "The Association Between Anemia and Postpartum Depression: A Systematic Review and Meta-Analysis," *Caspian Journal of International Medicine* 10, no. 2 (2019):115–124. doi: 10.22088/cjim.10.2.115.

13   J. Geohagan, D. de Gaston, A. Sadler, and P. Palmer, "Does Oral Maternal Vitamin D Supplementation Normalize the Vitamin D Level in Exclusively Breastfed Infants?" *Journal of the Oklahoma State Medical Association* 111, no. 10 (2018): 870–871.

14   A. M. Prentice, G. R. Goldberg, and A. Prentice, "Body Mass Index and Lactation Performance," *European Journal of Clinical Nutrition* 48 (1998) Suppl 3:S78–S89.

15   B. Kvenshagen, R. Halvorsen, and M. Jacobsen, "Adverse Reactions to Milk in Infants," *Acta Paediatrica* 97, no.2 (2008): 196–200. doi:10.1111/j.1651-2227.2007.00599.x.

16   R. F. Rodgers, J. L. O'Flynn, A. Bourdeau, and E. Zimmerman, "A Biopsychosocial Model of Body Image, Disordered Eating, and Breastfeeding Among Postpartum Women." *Appetite* 126, (2018):163–168. doi: 10.1016/j.appet.2018.04.007.

17   J. Linardon, L. Susanto, H. Tepper, and M. Fuller-Tyszkiewicz, "Self-Compassion as a Moderator of the Relationships Between Shape and Weight Overvaluation and Eating Disorder Psychopathology, Psychosocial Impairment, and Psychological Distress," *Body Image* 33 (2020):183–189. doi: 10.1016/j. bodyim.2020.03.001.

Acknowledgments

This book would not be possible without the love and support of my fiancé, who endured (and will continue to endure) countless conversations about hormones, birth, and postpartum. Thank you for cheering me on, and championing that all men should be feminist! To my daughter, Kaiya, who taught me about myself and ignited my passion for mothers everywhere. I love you eternally.

About the Author

Jaren Soloff is a registered dietitian and International Board-Certified Lactation Consultant (IBCLC) who serves as an expert in women's health. While continuing to practice in the field of eating disorder treatment, Jaren gained additional experience as an IBCLC to fuse her love of nutrition and women's health.

Now working solely in private practice, Jaren combines her expertise as a skilled nutrition therapist and lactation consultant to support individuals looking to heal their relationship with food and body. She created FULL CRCL (www.fullcrcl.co), which provides evidence-based practices to support women at all stages of the reproductive cycle, from preconception to postpartum. Informed by her own journey and the hundreds of women she has counseled, Jaren's experience comes full circle to support women in navigating pregnancy, birth, and postpartum from a simple and intuitive framework. You can find her chatting about all the women's health things on social media: @fullcrcl.